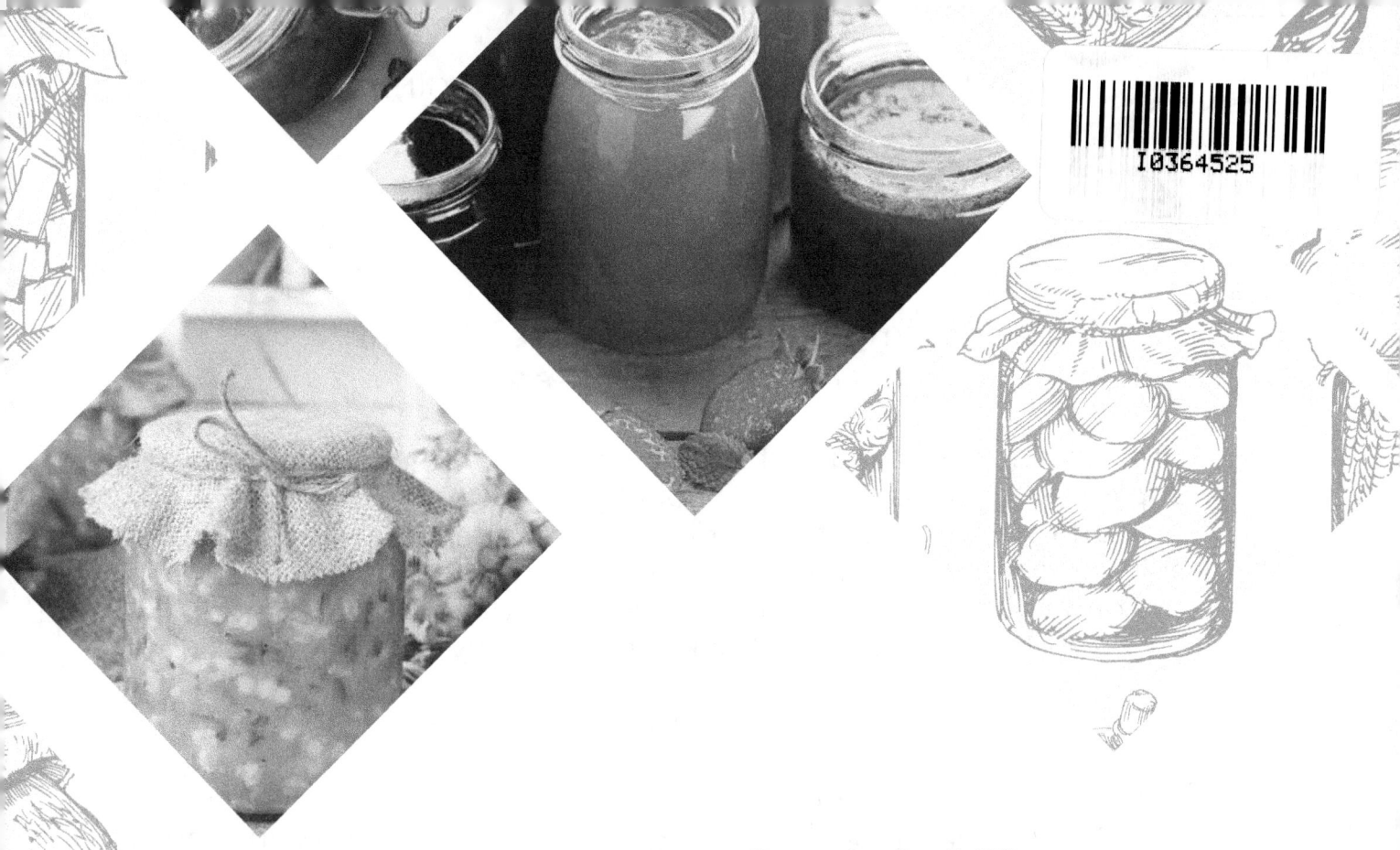

CANNING AND PRESERVING

FOR BEGINNERS

The Complete Guide to Can and Preserve Foods in Jars, with Easy and Tasty Recipes. Learn how to Preserve and Cook Veggies, Fruit, Meat, Poultry, Fish, and More.

VIVIAN BAYNE

Copyright - 2020 - by Vivian Bayne
All rights reserved.

The content contained within this book may not be reproduced, duplicated or transmitted without direct written permission from the author or the publisher. Under no circumstances will any blame or legal responsibility be held against the publisher, or author, for any damages, reparation, or monetary loss due to the information contained within this book. Either directly or indirectly.

Legal Notice:

This book is copyright protected. This book is only for personal use. You cannot amend, distribute, sell, use, quote or paraphrase any part, or the content within this book, without the consent of the author or publisher.

Disclaimer Notice:

Please note the information contained within this document is for educational and entertainment purposes only. All effort has been executed to present accurate, up to date, and reliable, complete information. No warranties of any kind are declared or implied. Readers acknowledge that the author is not engaging in the rendering of legal, financial, medical or professional advice. The content within this book has been derived from various sources. Please consult a licensed professional before attempting any techniques outlined in this book.

By reading this document, the reader agrees that under no circumstances is the author responsible for any losses, direct or indirect, which are incurred as a result of the use of information contained within this document, including, but not limited to, - errors, omissions, or inaccuracies.

TABLE OF CONTENTS

INTRODUCTION	7
CHAPTER 1.	
HISTORY AND DEVELOPMENT OF CANNING	11
CHAPTER 2.	
FAT TOM AND FOOD SAFETY	15
CHAPTER 3.	
MAIN PRESERVING METHODS	23
CHAPTER 4.	
PICKLING AND FERMENTING	29
CHAPTER 5.	
DEHYDRATING	33
CHAPTER 6.	
SMOKING	41
CHAPTER 7.	
CANNING AND PRESERVING TOOLS	45
CHAPTER 8.	
CANNING AND PRESERVING TIPS	51
CHAPTER 9.	
BENEFITS OF CANNING AND PRESERVING	59
CHAPTER 10.	
VEGETABLE RECIPES	63
1. Asparagus, Spears	67
2. Lima Beans, Shelled	68
3. White Potatoes: Cubed or Whole	69
4. Italian Style Stewed Tomatoes	70
5. Tomatoes: Whole	71
6. Spiced Beets	74

7. Spicy Carrots	75
8. Sweet Corn Salad	76
9. Garden Vegetable Medley	77
10. Mixed Vegetables, Italian Style	78

Chapter 11.
Meat and Poultry Recipes — 79

11. Dehydrated Candied Bacon	86
12. Soy Marinated Salmon Jerky	87
13. Teriyaki Beef Jerky	88
14. Pot Roast in a Jar	89
15. Canned Beef Stroganoff	90
16. Canned Ground Beef	91
17. Canned Chipotle Beef	92
18. Canned Goulash	93
19. Canned Chicken and Gravy	94
20. Canned Meatballs	95
21. Canned Pork	96
22. Canned Turkey	97
23. Canned Chili	98

Chapter 12.
Stock, Broths Soup and Stew Recipes — 99

24. Tomato Soup	104
25. Canned Mushroom Soup	105
26. Celery Soup	106
27. Navy Bean Soup	107
28. Carrot Soup	108
29. Taco Turkey Stew	109
30. Bean and Bacon Soup	110
31. Mexican Turkey Soup	111
32. Vegetarian Vegetable Soup	112
33. Canned Vegetable Soup	113
34. Pressure Canned Chicken Soup	114
35. Canned Carrot and Ginger Soup	115
36. Pressure Canned Tomato Soup	116
37. Canned Chicken Stock	117
38. American Chicken Stock	118
39. Home-Canned Beef Stock	119

40. Canned Turkey Stock — 120
41. Pressure Canned Turkey Broth — 121
42. Canned Beef Broth — 122
43. Pressure Canned Chicken Broth — 123
44. Pressure Canned Beef Stew — 124
45. Canned Hearty Chili Stew — 125
46. Canned Chili Con Carne — 126
47. Venison Stew with Veggies — 127

Chapter 13.
Full Meal Recipes — 129

48. Mashed Potatoes and Meatloaf — 130
49. Kielbasa and Sauerkraut — 131
50. Crockpot Chili — 132
51. Tuna Sandwiches — 133
52. Hearty Cowboy Trails Dinner — 134

Chapter 14.
Fruit, Juice, Jam & Jelly Recipes — 135

JAM
53. PINEAPPLE-RHUBARB JAM — 138
54. Honey Blueberry Cobbler Jam — 139
55. Canned Blueberry Jam — 140

CONSERVE
56. Victorian Plum Conserve — 141
57. Apple-Walnut Maple Conserve — 142

COMPOTE
58. Cranberry Pear Compote — 143
59. Delightful Fruit Compote — 144

MARMELADE
60. Quince Orange Marmalade — 145
61. Three-Fruit Marmalade — 146
62. Orange Pineapple Marmalade — 147
63. Pear Marmalade — 148
64. Tomato Lemon Marmalade — 149
65. Mixed Citrus Marmalade — 150

66. Strawberry Marmalade	**151**
67. Jalapeño Pepper Jelly	**152**
68. Just Jalapeno Blackberry Jelly	**153**
69. Savory Ruby Port Vinegar Jelly	**154**
70. Rosy Jelly Retreat	**155**
CONCLUSION	**157**
APPENDIX	**159**

INTRODUCTION

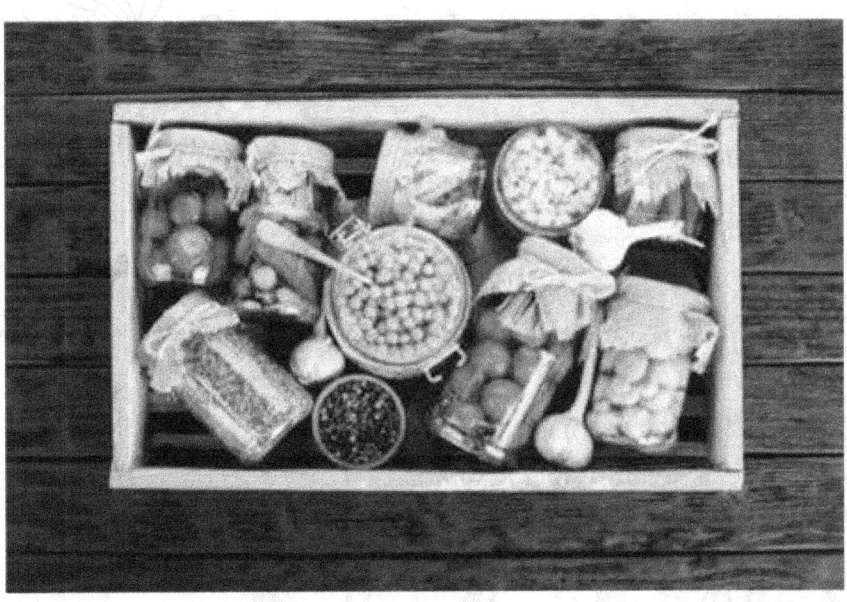

Have you ever pried open the lid of a store-bought can of soup, fruit, or vegetables and wished it contained the fresh flavors you wanted? More importantly, wouldn't it be nice to know what's really in your food without needing a dictionary? Canning and Preserving for Beginners gives you both of these things, without eating up all your free time. By applying the instructions in this book, anyone can create interesting, unique, preserved edibles at home that are spiced just right and created with love and care.

As you might suspect, this is not your run-of-the-mill recipe collection. From gourmet jam flavors and luscious mustards to mouthwatering marinades and pleasing pickles, you're going to find refreshingly creative recipes to add to your repertoire. Perhaps they'll even become new traditions. After entering the world of preserving, families will discover important budgetary advantages and the wonders of a full pantry that appeals to everyone's taste buds. Children will love helping out, and single readers will find that these methods can help with the not-wanting-to-cook-for-one-person blues. Now singles can preserve perfectly sized portions of a favorite creation and take out a single serving whenever the craving strikes.

Canning and Preserving for Beginners

It's true that the art of canning and preserving fell out of fashion for a while. After all, the supermarket had nearly anything you wanted at a reasonable cost. Today, things are different. What happened to inspire a renaissance? Many things. There's the move towards getting away from chemically treated food, and organic gardens have sprouted up in many backyards. This book is meant for anyone who wants to know what they put in their mouth is safe. It's also written for the large number of television viewers who have caught the cooking bug from various shows. Perhaps most important, more families are trying to find ways to protect valued histories, including recipes, and the art of preserving is one way of achieving that goal.

Beyond those three reasons, home preserving saves you money and fits in superbly with healthy living choices. With these methods, you can give your family the food they love, prepared the way you like it and neatly personalized for allergies or dietary restrictions! Better still, the endeavor isn't a one-shot deal; you end up with several months' worth of stock to enjoy. And you won't be alone in your efforts: Nearly 30 percent of Americans are rediscovering the natural goodness that canning and preserving offer.

If you're wondering whether you have the time or money for another hobby, don't worry. Canning and preserving doesn't require you to rework your kitchen to look like a magazine ad, and the cost of the basic components is more than covered by the savings in your grocery budget. It isn't even necessary to gather all the equipment for all preserving methods immediately. Instead, focus on one method and begin watching for bargains.

The book Canning and Preserving For Beginners, offers your kitchen tried-and-true methods for canning, freezing, drying, and pickling so you can pick what you like best. Additionally, throughout this book you'll find time-saving hints so you can really enjoy your projects. Food should be fun! Preserving is an alchemical art, and playing with your food is encouraged. While there are some guidelines you need to follow, there's still plenty of room for creativity. With that in mind, this book has one central underlying theme: Food changes life, life changes food, and preserving allows us to remember and celebrate this every day.

Canning and Preserving for Beginners

History shows that people try to develop food conservation techniques to preserve their food. You will find food preservation techniques from ancient times like salting, pickling, oil packing, fermentation, refrigeration under cool water, and smoking food to increase their shelf life.

Storing your own produce is a great way of dealing with the glut of fruits and vegetables any home grower will often experience. You will learn lots of different ways to store your produce, including some rather cool modern methods, plus lots and lots of recipes and ideas of what to make with your vegetables.

The book contains modern food canning and preservation techniques that guide you on how to preserve your food using water bath canning and the pressure canning method. Canning is one of today's most popular and advanced food preservation techniques used to preserve vegetables, fruits, soups, meat, dairy product, syrup, juices, and jellies. Canning is one of the thermal processes in which all kinds of microorganisms are destroyed and the food is sealed into an airtight container. Instead of a glass jar, most of the modern vacuum techniques use aluminum, steel, plastic, and glass containers for sealing purposes. These containers are reused again and again during this method. Canning is the perfect way to preserve your favorite food with more than a year-long shelf life. It means that in summer fresh blueberry is canned and used in winter without changing the taste, texture, and color of food.

This book guides you and helps you to know more about canning from basics. It also contains useful tips for water bath canning and pressure canning. The book comes with delicious and tasty canning recipes. These recipes are written with their exact preparation, cooking time, and their exact nutritional value information. All the recipes written in this book are unique and written in a simple understandable form.

FOLLOW USDA-APPROVED RECIPES

Canning and preserving should be done in a proper way to prevent unnecessary health hazards/risks. Ensure that you always follow USDA-approved recipes as they will contain everything you need to know, including up-to-date safety measures. USDA-approved recipes provide adequate salt ratios, preparation guidance, and storage measures for pickling or fermenting foods. Avoid heritage recipes that may lack proper safety standards to avoid botulism or other types of potentially fatal food poisoning.

The USDA has lists of certified recipes that are known for following proper, modern safety measures to ensure that you are using the best recipes possible. Understand that heritage recipes may have worked for people in the past, but those people did not know what we know now. As a result, many of them fell ill from consuming their food. These days, we have access to proper research, science, and technology that allows us to safely preserve and store foods without risking our health, or the health of our family. If you do choose to use a heritage recipe, compare it to the USDA standards and adjust it as needed, to ensure that your recipe is safe for use. The recipes in this book follow USDA approved guidelines, but you should always keep yourself updated by checking the USDA site:

https://nchfp.uga.edu/publications/publications_usda.html

Chapter 1.
History and Development of Canning

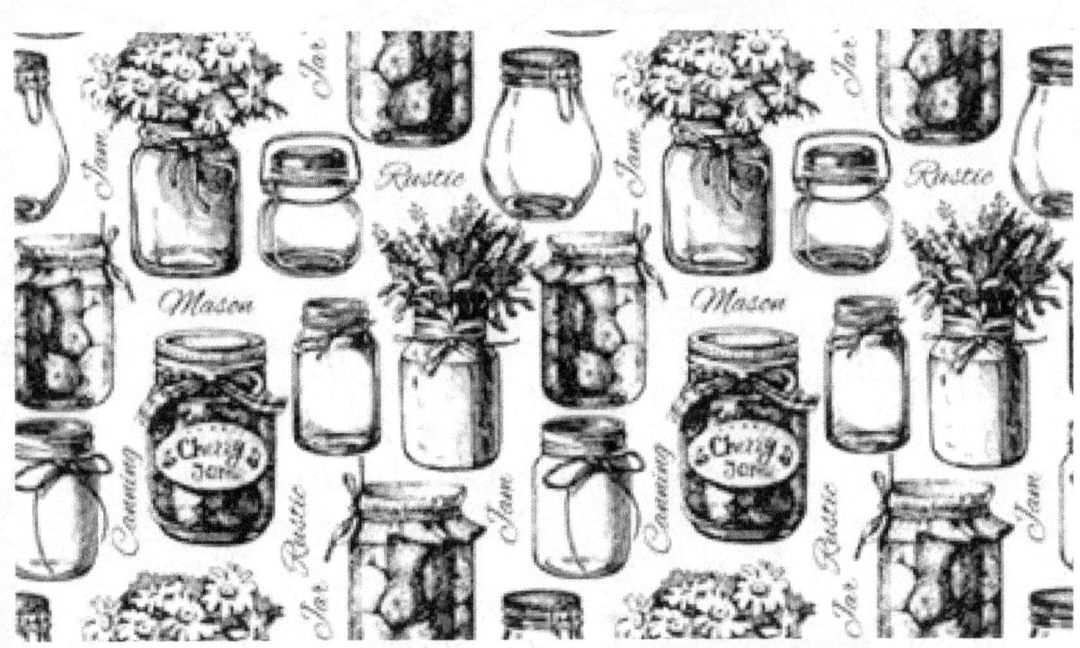

The need to preserve food dates as far back as the first years of the Napoleonic Wars. The French government offered the hefty reward of 12,000 francs to the inventor that could produce an effective way of preserving large quantities of food for a prolonged period of time. The requirement resulted from the need to support Napoleon's military campaigns. The winner of the contest was Nicolas Appert in 1809.

He noticed that unless the seals leaked, the food cooked inside a jar did not spoil. Acting on this observation he developed a method to seal food in glass jars. The reason that the food did not spoil, was discovered 50 years later by none other than Louis Pasteur who noticed and recorded how microbes affected the food spoilage. Glass jars presented a challenge, as there were a lot of problems involved in their transportation. The solution was given by Peter Durand in 1810 who devised the familiar cylindrical wrought-iron canisters (the root of the modern term cans). Durand's cans solved the fragility problem of the glass jars and they were also cheaper and faster to manufacture. However, glass jars still remain as a good option for canning high value products at home.

Durand's cans may have solved the glass jars' inadequacies, but they presented another problem. Not everyone could use a bayonet to open a can up. Sometimes it was necessary to smash the cans with rocks to open them up. This necessitated the development of a can opener which didn't happen until 1840, largely due to the fact that the factory and the know-how of Nicolas Appert were all but destroyed in 1814 by the coalition soldiers invading France.

The next step was the development of the famous tin can. It would seem that the entire canning concept was something that the French could be identified with (in a similar fashion that the Fins were identified with driving and the Brazilians identified with soccer), as another Frenchman, Philippe de Girard was the one who thought of the method and developed it with the assistance of Bryan Donkin and John Hall. The product was dubbed as a tin can because the material used was tinned wrought iron.

Tin cans became a massive success. Initially amongst the military forces of the British Army and the Royal Navy and then commercially. It is indicative of this success that by the mid-19th century, canned food became a status symbol for the middle class.
This success was mitigated heavily after the Franklin expedition disaster in 1845, which vividly demonstrated that canned food may entail serious health hazards. In this case it was the lead solder that was used for sealing the cans and that was proved to be extremely poisonous to humans. The situation was remedied through various improvements and side inventions, and by 1860 the increase in urban populations demanded for increasing quantities of canned food. At that point, the time required to cook food in a sealed can was reduced from six hours to thirty minutes.

The next major advancement in the canning technology occurred during World War I. In the beginning the food contained was cheap and of low quality. The majority of the cans contained the then famous 'Bully Beef' which was actually very cheap corned beef. To improve the morale of their soldiers the British begun purchasing food of higher quality and then created the staple of all military forces even to this date: the complete meals.

As incredible as it may seem, the last major development that occurred around the 1900s remains the same until today. And this is the double seeming technique which completely sealed the cans and made them totally airtight and allowed for the food inside to remain uncompromised for a period of at least five years, even at the worst of storing conditions.

The only change that has happened during the manufacturing stage of a can recently, is the substitution of steel and wrought iron with aluminum compounds, which made the can production faster and cheaper.

While it is possible to manufacture metal cans at home, it is preferable to either purchase readily made ones that have observed the safety precautions, or use glass jars if you want to prepare and can your own canned food and keep it stored to be used in case of an emergency.

CANNING TODAY

Nowadays, people can and preserve for various reasons. Even with all the industrial preserving methods at their all-time best, most of us like the idea of canning and preserving our own foods in the comfort of our homes.

This is done for several reasons:

- Industrial methods of preservation have grown unhealthier for our bodies in the long term and can cause many diseases with prolonged use.
- Many people have made a hobby out of canning and preserving and like to gift friends with their wonderful combinations as a rustic gift.
- It's much safer to can and preserve using new methods like pressure canning and water bath methods.
- Equipment and tools are easily available to preserve your own jams,

sauces, dry spices, and other foods.
- *Now you can preserve the vegetables and fruits that you love that aren't available all year around.*
- *This is an eco-friendly way of recycling. Mason jars are reusable, and by canning your own food you can help reduce industrial waste.*
- *You can preserve personal harvest using these methods and save the food for later, or for gifting others.*
- *The quality and taste of your own pickled and canned foods is unparalleled and can't be compared to store bought canned items.*

Chapter 2.
FAT TOM and Food Safety

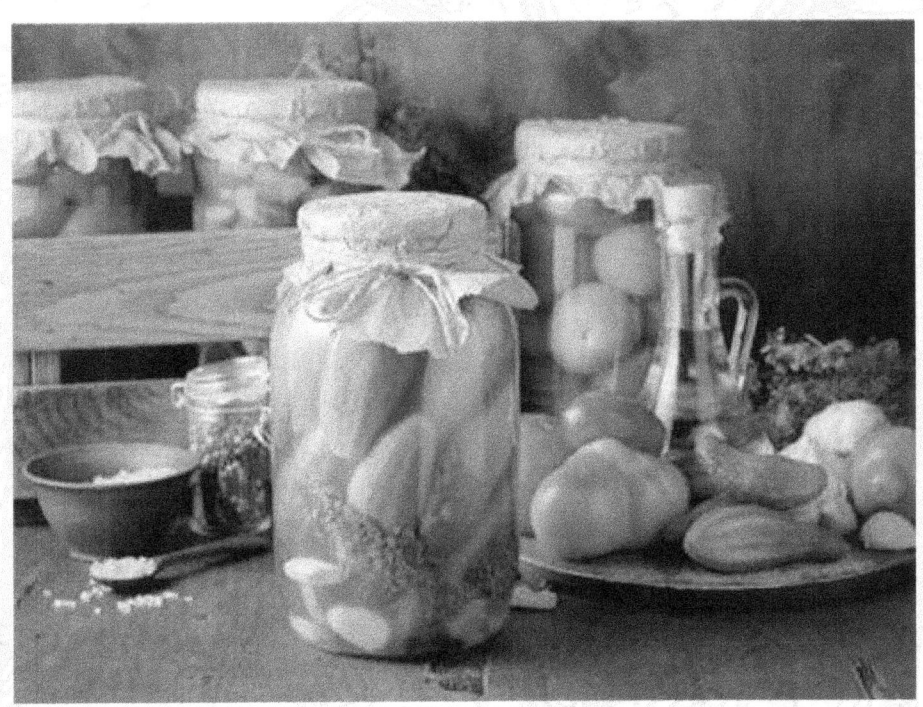

In this book you will discover the most common canning and preserving techniques and learn how to use them to cook easy and tasty recipes. Before starting to get into action though, let's learn some of the basics about food safety and have a quick look at the main factors that contribute to food spoilage.

Whatever canning and preserving method you decide to use, you should always consider and try to prevent the risks involved with handling and preserving food. There is an easy mnemonic device that can help with it: FAT TOM (to remember it, you may think of a big guy named Tom).

These are the 6 factors:

F - FOOD (PARTICLES, ETC.)

Living microorganisms (bacteria, yeast, and mold) are a natural part of our existence. They are all around us, including in the air we breathe. Some have health benefits that have led us to produce lifesaving antibiotics (like penicillin) and other medicines, yet others can cause foods to spoil or lead to serious illness. When working with food in the kitchen, we must concern ourselves with harmful pathogenic microorganisms like staphylococcus and salmonella, which cause food-borne illnesses, and we must learn how to prevent them from invading our food source.

With any living thing, certain conditions are required for optimal growth. The perfect environment for harmful pathogenic microorganisms is moisture, between 60 °F and 90 °F, and an environment that has available free oxygen. However, while those are prime conditions, microorganisms can grow in temperatures as low as 40 °F and as high as 140 °F. So be mindful of those leftovers that you kept lying out on the countertop; there is a reason we push to get them refrigerated, below 40 °F, as soon as possible.

So how does canning prevent harmful microorganisms from invading our food? With proper food preparation, like scrubbing the exterior of root crops, knowledge of a recipe's overall pH, and the application of high heat and adequate processing times, the dangerous bacteria will not survive in a sealed jar of food. Let's take a closer look at common food spoilers:

BACTERIA

One of the most predominate bacterium associated with home canning is Clostridium botulinum, known to produce a toxin that causes a disease called 'Botulism.' While some harmful microorganisms require oxygen to grow and multiply, this particular bacterium requires an anaerobic environment, or an environment without free oxygen. This makes a sealed jar of food a perfect environment, but it's only perfect if the bacterium is present to begin with. That is why it is imperative to thoroughly wash vegetables and properly handle meat and fish when canning. Also, following proper processing methods is the key to killing this harmful bacterium in the event that it escapes thorough cleaning and makes its way into the jar.

ENZYMES

Enzymes are natural proteins found in plants and animals that speed up chemical reactions. They are also responsible for the ripening of fruits and vegetables. Ironically, the enzymes that make our food ready to eat are the same enzymes that cause our food to spoil if not eaten within a suitable time frame. Why? These enzymes stay active even after produce is harvested and meat is slaughtered. So how do we prevent our food from spoiling? We expose it to acid and/or high heat.

MOLDS AND YEASTS

Molds are microscopic fungi that live on plant and animal matter. There are thousands of species that produce spores. Spores float through the air undetected and can also be transported by water and insects. A poorly sealed jar is the perfect place for spores to take root and grow. The roots may be difficult to see, as they may start very deep within the food, but the mold is visible as it grows and produces streaks of colors and then fuzz. Yeast spores grow on food much in the same way mold spores do, preferring acidic and sugary foods, like pickles and jam.

When preparing fruits and vegetables to preserve, discard any foods with fuzzy mold or slimy goo. You cannot just cut off the mold or try to wash off the slime. Mold and yeast are impervious to acid. The only way to destroy mold spores and yeast when canning is to expose them to high heat for a specific period of time.

Learning your way around all the tools that are used for canning can be awe-inspiring and intimidating.

FOODS THAT YOU CAN CAN

When you're thinking about canning, you'll want to can things like:

- Fruits
- Vegetables
- Fruit Juices
- Pickles
- Jams
- Relishes
- Condiments

- Jellies
- Vinegars
- Salsas
- Chutneys
- Poultry
- Meat
- Fish

FOODS THAT YOU CANNOT CAN

There are some foods that you will not be able to can such as:

- Flour products, whey, and oats
- Dairy Soy, and Fats
- Thickeners
- Mashed Veggies
- High-Fat Meats
- Candies

These ingredients tend to not work well with the canning process and can go bad inside of the can.

A - ACIDITY (PH)

The pH scale goes from 0 to 14, with 0 being the most basic or least acidic, and 14 being the most acidic. Adding a little bit of lemon juice helps the pectin gel as it should.
However, if your fruit and or vegetable has a starting pH above 4.6, it cannot be processed with water bath canning (you will need a pressure canner) until the pH is lowered to 4.6 or below. So, to lower the pH just add in some bottled lime or lemon juice to your fruit, and then measure the pH. Perhaps you are wondering why pH matters. Well if the pH is above 4.6, it can be unsafe to eat any jams or jellies made thereof, as bacteria thrives in a sealed jar at those low acid pH levels. Also, you want to understand the pH of your food to discover how you can achieve a good balance of flavors. Acidity or sourness are as essential as salt or seasoning to yield a well-balanced meal. Using bottled lemon or lime juice is the safest way to reduce the pH, as it is often the most consistent and tested product.

HOW DO I MEASURE THE PH?

You can rest assured that the recipes in this book have been kitchen tested and are below pH 4.6, therefore safe to cook. You won't need to measure the pH of your food.
If, however you are curious and wondering how you could measure the pH of food, you need to know that there are mainly two ways to do it:

- By litmus paper (also referred to as pH test strips) where you dip the paper strip into a solution and compare the color to a reference chart. This method may be prone to inaccuracy, as it relies on the ability of the human eye to match the color on the strip to the reference chart. It is also dependent on the temperature of the food (most strips are standardized at 77 °F or 25 °C) and it might not be 100% accurate.
- By a pH meter and electrode. This is a more accurate and less prone to mistakes method. My recommendation is not to buy the cheapest tool on the market but look for one that is good enough to be reliable and last long. You will also need a calibration solution (not cheap either), some distilled water (you can find it in any pharmacy store for a reasonable price) and an electrode, that should be replaced from time to time. A pH meter requires good care in terms of calibration, cleaning and storing, to ensure its accuracy over time.

As mentioned, if you follow USDA approved and tested recipes, you may never have to worry about your food pH.

T - TIME (EXPOSURE DURATION AT DIFFERENT TEMPERATURES)

Food should be removed from "the danger zone" within two to four hours. This can be done either by cooling or heating. See the next section for more information about the "danger zone".

T - TEMPERATURE (REFERS TO 'DANGER ZONE')

Pathogens in food grow best in temperatures between 41 to 135 °F (5 to 57 °C). This is called the temperature danger zone (TDZ). Food-borne pathogens thrive in temperatures that are between 70 to 104 °F (21 to 40 °C).

The food is preserved in canned jars when agents that cause spoilage are destroyed with heat, and by getting rid of air out of the food, and also sealing jars to prevent yeast, air, bacteria and molds from being introduced again in the food.

Four Reasons Why Foods Spoil

- Yeasts are killed at 140 °F – 190 °F.
- Enzymes are killed at 140 °F.
- Molds are killed at 140 °F – 190 °F.
- Bacteria: These along with related toxins are destroyed at 190 °F – 240 °F.

Bear in mind that when canned non-acidic or low-acidic foods are boiled for 10-20 minutes prior to consuming them, this can destroy any toxin that are likely to be lingering. When you do this, you will have an additional cause for feeling safe about consuming home canned foods that do not have any acid or have low acid levels.

O - OXYGEN (AEROBIC, ANAEROBIC)

In order to avoid consuming canned foods which are not good anymore and which can be harmful to health, toss out jars showing warning signs. When there is a convex lid, it means that the container that the food is in was not properly sealed. There is a great possibility that the jar is overstuffed or broken if the liquid is leaking out of the jar. There may be fermentation, or the food is past the due date, if the liquid spurts out when the jar is opened. If there is an unnatural odor coming from your canned food, do not hesitate to toss it into the garbage.

BACTERIA

There are several kinds of bacteria. Some bacteria are produced by the toxins that are also dangerous. There are some very tough bacteria that are hard to die even when the temperatures are high.

Clostridium Botulinum

The toughest of these is the Clostridium botulinum, which results in a dangerous illness that affects the nervous system. This illness is known as botulism. This anaerobic organism thrives in conditions with low oxygen like a jar or can that is not properly sealed.

Heat range of 190 °F can kill the bacterium, and 240 °F can destroy the toxic spores.

The bacterium lives and flourishes in foods that have low-acid levels or no acid at all, when there is no air present. The foods that can be included in this group include meat, poultry, fish, beans, peppers, beans and corn. For this reason, it is highly important that these kinds of foods are given high pressure during the canning process.

M - MOISTURE (WATER ACTIVITY)

Fresh food is comprised of between 10 and 30 % air. The quality of your food depends on how much is removed during processing. Raw food should be packed using the hot packing method.

Hot packing involves prepared, but unheated food. This is especially true with fruit. The air that is trapped around the food will cause discoloration in a period of 2 to 3 months.

Hot packing involves heating food to the boiling point and allowing it to simmer for only 2 to 3 minutes. Pack the food into jars at the boiling temperature. This will prevent air from staying in the jar, keep fruit from floating, and improve the shelf time of the food.

At first, the hot pack method may leave the fruit looking no different than the raw pack method, but after being in storage for a while, you will notice the difference.

Always follow the directions in a recipe, even if it tells you to raw pack, as they have all been tried and proven.

ALTITUDE ADJUSTMENTS

It is always possible to find a regional cookbook that has already figured out altitude adjustments, but this is highly unusual. Every book I have seen assumes you are at or near sea level. Why is this important? Because altitude affects the temperature, at which water boils. If you live below 1,000 feet above sea level, you have no corrections to make to the process.

If you live between 1,000 and 2,000 feet above sea level, you need to begin making adjustments. There is no need to adjust pressure canning, yet, but if using water bath canning, an adjustment is needed. When above 2,000 feet, adjustments are needed to be made in pressure canning.

Pressure canning requires no change in the processing time, but does require changes for the pressure to be held at, so that the temperature inside the canner reaches 240 °F. This temperature is what kills the botulism bacteria. More information about this can found in the pressure canning details.

Chapter 3.
Main Preserving Methods

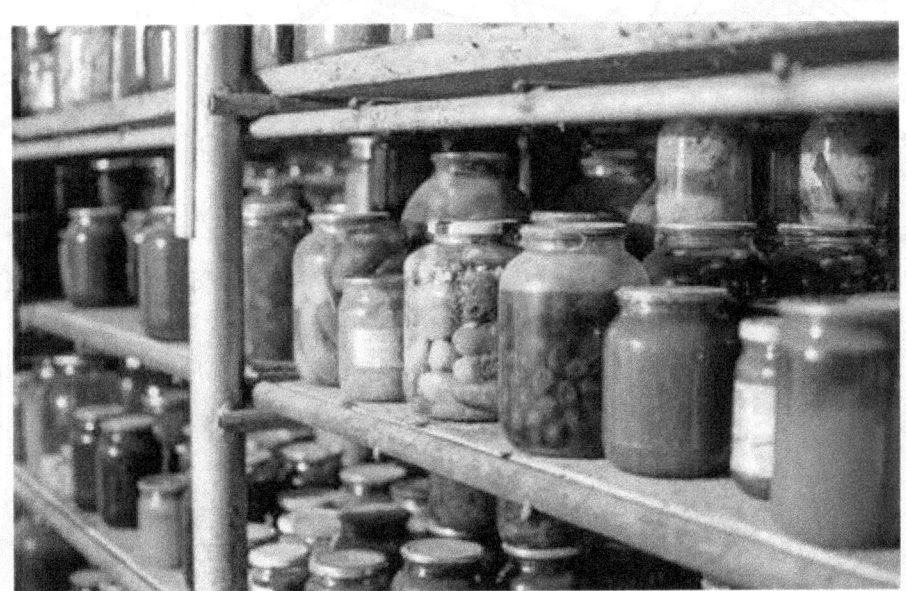

Canning and preserving are terms that are often interchanged with one another. Basically, both refer to techniques that involve putting food in containers for a longer shelf life.

CANNING

Canning is a preservation technique that involves heating food to a high temperature to attenuate harmful microorganisms that cause the food to spoil, as well as health problems to people. During the canning method, the food inside the container is heated at extremely high temperatures that result in air being driven out from the can, thereby creating a vacuum seal as the container cools. The absence of air improves the shelf-life of food and prevents it from being re-contaminated by microorganisms.

WATER BATHING

Water bathing is the most popular form of processing for many canners.

Water bath canning is for acidic foods such as jams, salsas, and pickles that only require a boiling water temperature (212 °F or 100 °C at sea level) to safely kill harmful bacteria. . Water bathing requires a large stockpot or canner and a jar rack to prevent jars from clanking into each other and cracking. Water completely covers every jar and is heated to a full rolling boil to ensure that you have attained 212 °F. Jars are then processed for the specific amount of time indicated in the recipe.

Because only high-acid foods can be processed in a hot water bath, we can rely on the temperature of boiling water to safely preserve the food. This means, however, that the jars must be adequately covered with water and the water must be at a full rolling boil for the entire processing time to ensure that the required 212 °F temperature penetrates the contents of each jar. If any of the jars are exposed to air (not covered by water), it is likely that harmful bacteria will grow in the portion of exposed food. It is not recommended to water bathe low-acid foods because, given the length of time required to do it so safely (upwards of 3 hours), it is very tricky to ensure that each jar stays covered with water and the water is kept at a consistent 212 °F for the full length of processing.

PRESSURE CANNING

A regulated technique of preserving foods, such as fruits and vegetables with a pressure canner or pressure cooker, which is used for the cooking and heating process is called pressure canning. Food contents are being placed in separate jars and evenly set collectively in the pressure pot that contains water. In order to produce steam that sterilizes, cooks, and seals the food airtight in the jars, the contents are heated under pressure to a very high temperature. As it rises in the canner, the warm steam passes through the food with force, to cook and preserve it meticulously. Pressure canning is a common method of preserving vegetables, fish, poultry, meats, fruits, and other edibles.

PRESSURE CANNERS

The pressure canner is ideal for canning low-acid vegetables, meats, and beans. A temperature of 240 °F is required to kill bacteria in these foods. Pressure canners use steam to push all the air out of the canner. The steam and the water in the canner combine to reach the high temperatures required to kill harmful bacteria. These canners have both electric and non-electronic models. It is recommended by the USDA to find a pressure canner large enough to hold at least 4-quart of the jars. A pressure canner is no less expensive than the water bath container, ranging from $75 - $300 in price. The only difference is that a pressure canner can do the work of both canners. Ultimately, for effective canning you want to have both options, depending on what you plan to can. Pressure canners also have two types, the dial gauge and the weight gauge. These both indicate and regulate the pressure in the canner, but the dial gauge pressure canners are probably your best bet, even though they're about $20 more expensive than the weight gauge.

Dial Gauge: In addition to the dial gauge itself, these canners will have a counterweight that you place onto the open vent pipe to pressurize the canner. While processing, you simply refer to the recipe for pressure and weight specifics. The recipe will state the proper number to reach on the gauge (10 or something, for example), as well as tell you the counterweight setting for the little weight you place the air vent. These two elements work together to process the food properly.

REFRIGERATION AND FREEZING

Refrigeration and freezing are common everyday household techniques that enable food to be kept for longer. If refrigeration is slowing down the growth of microorganisms, then freezing is magnifying this process. It is particularly useful to prolong the quality of foods that have been prepared or cooked already, but perhaps in their original forms they may not have required the refrigeration or freezing process. For example, potatoes do not require refrigeration or freezing to preserve them but cooked into a rösti or waffle, they do.

SUGARING

Sugar is a preservative and has typically been used to preserve fruit. Similar to salt, it draws moisture away so microorganisms cannot thrive. It is typically used in a syrup form and fruit is allowed to sit in it, keeping it for longer, particularly peeled fruit, or the fruit can be heated with the sugar.

SALTING

Salting is a subcategory of the drying method. Similar to drying, salt draws out the water in meats. Some salt curing processes add sugar for the same effect.

CURING

Just like salting, curing also involves the use of salt. However, aside from salt, it also makes use nitrites and other seasonings that should be applied to the meat. Essentially, you just soak the meat in a solution that contains salts and all the other ingredients, and doing so does not only preserve the meat, but also makes it taste better. After applying these ingredients and soaking the meat, you just have to let your meat sit for several hours until the moisture within has already been drawn out.

NATURAL CONSERVATION

Natural preservation is the best technique for storing vegetables. How? Wash thoroughly, cut and place in the sterilized jars in the case of raw vegetables and wash, cut and boil in salted water before placing in the jars in the case of cooked vegetables.

PRESERVATION IN OIL

Preservation in oil uses extra virgin olive oil to preserve mushrooms, spring onions and artichokes for a long time. The main thing is to put them in a dry jar, do not leave empty spaces and check that the oil covers the vegetables.

JELLYING

There are a variety of items that create a jelly-type base for preserving, including fruit pectin, gelatin, and arrowroot flour. After jellying, the resulting food is often canned for increased longevity.

JUICING

Basically, juicing is the process of breaking down your food and extracting the juice that it contains. The most common types of food that are being juiced are fruits and vegetables. In this process, you just have to liquefy all the parts of the fruit or vegetable so that you can get all the vitamins, minerals, as well as fiber that comes with it. You can extract the juice from the fruit or vegetables by either using the pressure of your hand or using automatic juicers. In this process, you can make use of different types of juicers such as blender juicers, centrifugal juicers, masticating juicers, and many more.

You can consume the juice either raw or cooked. Many experts say, however, that drinking the juice raw is better since it still contains all the natural nutrients from the fruit or vegetables in which it was extracted from. But you can also include the juice to some of your dishes to make them healthier and much tastier.

Chapter 4.
Pickling and Fermenting

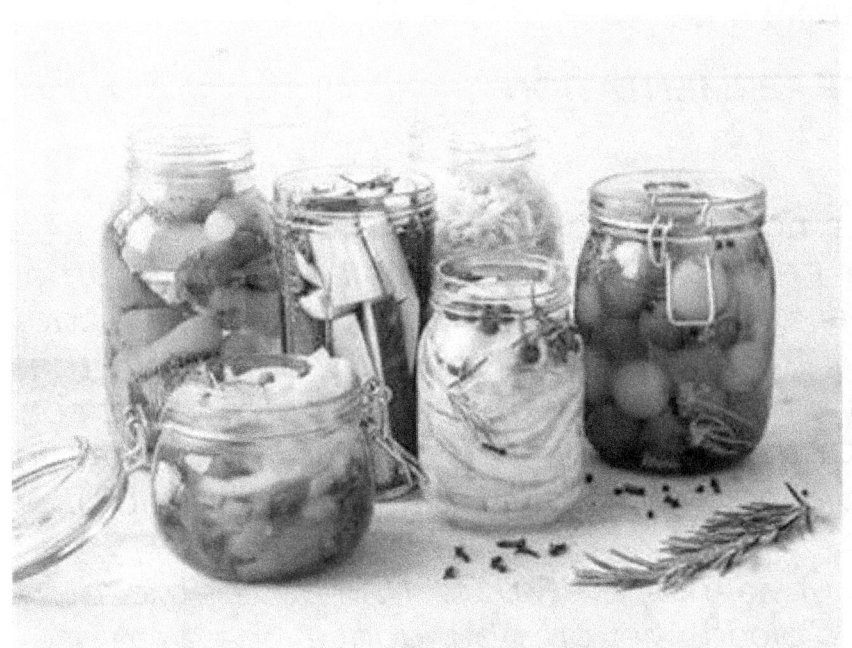

Pickling is a culinary art that people of different cultures practice all over the globe. To give you an idea what pickled foods look like, examples include, kosher cucumber pickles, salsas, pickled herring, chutneys, kimchi, miso pickles, and others. These examples are found in different countries, and that goes to underline the fact that pickling is a global practice. The big question, really, is what you do in order to be able to say you have pickled your food.

To make pickles or to pickle your food, what you do is to dip it in a solution that ensures the food has a long shelf life. Salting food is another complementary way of ensuring your food can last long without getting spoilt.

In ancient times, nomadic tribes of Africa and elsewhere would salt their meat to ensure it lasts many days and sometimes weeks. In fact, people of different cultures would preserve their food supplies for use during the winter season or during famine, and for that *lengthy preservation they would do salting and pickling. Sometimes people use vinegar for pickling, and this is because vinegar is acidic enough to kill bacteria that would otherwise cause food to go bad. Other foods are pickled in salt brine, and that is because it is a liquid that enhances fermentation. The reason fermentation is encouraged here is that good bacteria ends up developing, and that makes the food much less vulnerable to the bad bacteria. And, of course, if the growth of bad bacteria is restricted, it means your food cannot get spoilt quickly.*

BENEFITS OF FERMENTATION
HEALTH

First and foremost, let us take a look into the science of fermentation, and how it is beneficial for the human body. It is common knowledge that microbes and bacteria can be good as well as bad. In truth, the human body has evolved over millions of years in the company of microbes, and hence, has established a harmonious connection with them. In fact, there are approximately 10 trillion cells in the human body, but our bodies have almost 10 times that number of bacterial cells!

Microbes occupy almost every part of our bodies, except muscle tissues, the brain, and blood. They are abundant everywhere else. While it may seem disturbing to have all of these organisms on us and inside of us, they are vital for life! They provide us with vitamins and minerals; they create an environment unsuitable to harmful microbes by basically taking over all the nutrients or altering the environment; they regulate the functions of our digestive tracts, and help to fortify our immune systems.

The immune system has one of the most complex process of triggers, responses, chemicals, and signals in our bodies. We are being constantly attacked by microbes looking for a new host to proliferate in. They attack via air, food, and water. They are devious and will set themselves up anywhere they can find a suitable environment. For that reason, our friendly microbes act as impediments to harmful microbes.

MICROBES

Since this book focuses on food, we should discuss the major microbes in our digestive systems. Our intestines host the most widespread populations of microbes in the body. They are divided into four groups, but the intestinal microbes serve as more than just guards: they also play very important roles in our daily lives.

The four main types of intestinal microbes are:

1. Bifidobacteria
2. Lactobacilli
3. Ingested microbes
4. Fungi

The first two groups are vital for good health, while the ingested microbes are usually harmful. And the fungi, like yeast and mold, can be beneficial or harmful, depending on their numbers and strains. Bifidobacteria consists of around thirty species found widely in the digestive system (as well as other places). They help thwart pathological (harmful) bacteria from colonizing the gut. They also regulate and strengthen the immune system. Many fermented foods are rich in Bifidobacteria, and hence, great for health. Additionally, fermentation has also been shown to terminate or decrease certain compounds that are injurious to our health, including pesticide residue.

FLAVOR

One major reason to ferment vegetables is instantly evident with your first bite: the taste! Fermentation lives in a kingdom of food science that can seem like magic. These flavors are difficult, if not impossible, to duplicate without fermentation. That is one reason why great chefs all over the world love fermentation.

FUN AND EASE

Fermentation is for everyone. You don't need to be a professional cook to make fermented vegetables, although the flavors that this process creates will have your friends and family thinking that you are. If you can slice a vegetable, you can ferment it. Follow just a few basic *and flexible guidelines, and you'll have never ending fun fermenting vegetables to your heart and gut's content.*

Chapter 5.
Dehydrating

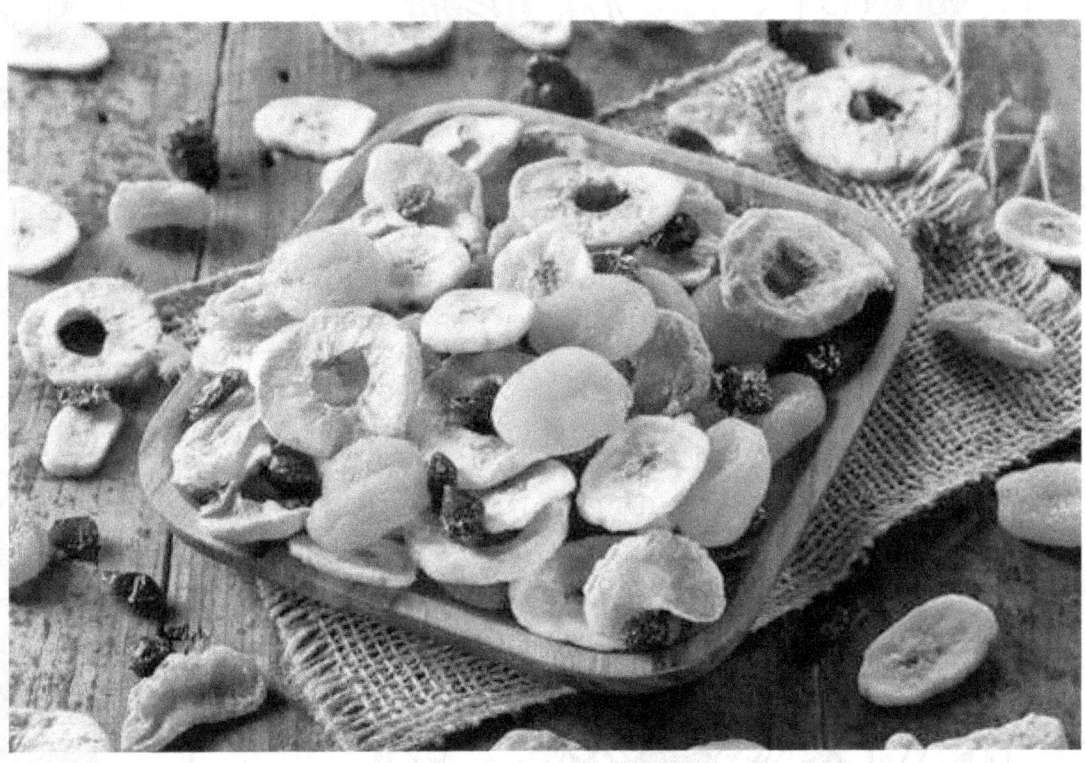

Dehydration which is popularly known as 'drying' is a long-practiced method for preserving foods. It can also be referred as the process of removing water through evaporation from a solid or liquid food. The aim of this is to arrive at a solid material that has been sufficiently water-reduced. This process consists of reducing the level of food moisture into smaller levels in order to extend the lifespan of the food. It requires adding different forms of energy to the food.

Note that dehydration does not include mechanical pressing of liquid foods. In most cases, Hot-air is used to add heat to the food and to reduce its moisture.

It is very easy for pathogenic bacteria to survive comfortably in the unfavorable environment of dried foods. This means that once your dried food is rehydrated and eaten, it could cause you food poisoning. Of course, you would not want to suffer food poisoning, all in the name of preserving your foods for later use.

What should you do then to prevent this when drying your food? Make use of high-quality materials with low contaminants when drying your foods. High-quality materials with low contaminants are materials and tools specifically made for dehydrating foods. Also, ensure proper sanitation of all tools and surfaces and ensure that the storage condition of the dried food is one that prevents contact with dust, rodents, insects and other house insects.

When you decide to dehydrate your food to make it last longer, then you have numerous options available for you. You could dry your food by air, vacuum, inert gas, steaming, or by directly applying heat to the food. Usually, the most popular and acceptable means of drying is by air. This is okay for obvious reasons. Using this method allows your food to dry gradually, plus it is very convenient. And, yes, air is very plentiful, and free! Allowing your food to dry gradually by using air prevents scorching and discoloration of your food, which is popular with other drying systems.

Dehydrating foods started as far back as times when early men spread their harvests or hunts out in the sun for sun drying. It is one of the oldest methods of preservation, as the prehistoric men were fond of drying some seeds before planting.

Fish, meats and food plants have been preserved over the years by drying them in the sun or naturally spreading them in the desert heat, across different desert areas.

In more recent times, American Indians stored their meats by laying them under the sun. The people of China also dried their eggs from the sunshine and the Japanese dried rice and fish under the sun's rays as well. During the Second World War, there was a great need to move food in bulk from place to place and this challenge ignited the developments of modern strategies on preserving foods, hence dehydration. In the year 1975 however, the French made a major breakthrough in the development of hot-air dehydration, which is the drying of foods through the method of blowing hot air over them.

THE PROCESS

Food dehydration involves the following processes;

1. The simultaneous transfer of mass and heat around the food.
2. A medium used to transfer energy around the food.
3. In the absence of hot-air, food dehydration can also be practiced through the use of other gases that can help reduce the moisture in the food.

THE OBJECTIVES OF FOOD DEHYDRATION

- Impacting a peculiar feature, such as a different crispiness and flavor, to a food product: An example is the transformation of maize to cereal.
- Shrinking the food material into smaller and more portable sizes to change their forms: Food materials, when the water has been reduced, become more portable and are easily packaged for transportation. Examples are the draining and grinding of curry leaves, thymes seeds etc. into spices.
- Reducing the volume and the weight of the food: The volume of water poses a substantial addition to the volume and weight of the food, by reducing the water content, the weight and volume of the food particle is also reduced.
- The conversion of food meals to a different form that is more convenient for storage, packaging and easy transportation: A great example is the conversion of milk or dairies to dry powder. When these products get to the places of consumption, they are reconverted to the previous forms through the addition of water.
- The effect of water depression which leads to preservation and longevity of the nutrients.

ADVANTAGES AND DISADVANTAGES OF DEHYDRATION

There are several advantages of dehydrating food, although all food storage processes also have their disadvantages. We shall briefly examine some of these advantages and disadvantages.

ADVANTAGES

1. *Extended Lifespan:* When foods are dehydrated, they last longer because the moisture is reduced and the dry food does not encourage the survival of bacteria. The absence of bacteria keeps food in good shape and this can last for as long as three months. When food items are dehydrated, they are sometimes converted into substances that can last a lifetime. Examples are spices such as cinnamon and curry powder which is derived from the dehydration and grinding of curry leaves. In most cases, spices like this can last for several years without getting spoiled.
2. *Waste Reduction:* When foods spoil, they reduce the amount of food available for consumption. Some food preservative methods usually give a very short extension before the spoilage of food. In many cases when we buy raw materials in the markets, the ability and knowledge to store them in good conditions help us keep the foods for a long time.
3. *Improvement in Food Taste:* The application of heat to reduce the water tastes in foods brings out the original taste of the other constituents of the food. The process of dehydration greatly improves the taste of food. When foods are water-filled, they are sometimes tasteless or acrid. When fruits are dried, the real taste is felt. In most cases, food tastes better when they are dehydrated.
4. *Easy Storage:* The fact that dehydrating foods make them easy to be stored is a great advantage of the process. When large bulks of foods are preserved in smaller packages, like the case of milk dehydrated into powder, it aids transportation and storekeeping. Through dehydration, storage is easier as it takes up lesser spaces.
5. *Preservation of Nutrients:* Dehydrating food maintains the nutrients in the food before they are dehydrated. Nutrients such as minerals, vitamins and enzymes are absolutely preserved during dehydration. Dehydration is the only method that can ascertain the preservation of nutrients in food particles. Cooking and other preservative methods often lead to loss of nutrients. The entire essence of consuming food is to get benefits from the nutrients, if these nutrients are reduced; the essence of consuming the food has been lost.
6. *Absence of Chemicals:* The only substance needed to dehydrate food is the heat added to the food material. Unlike some other preservative methods, it does not involve the addition of chemicals. Dehydrating

food therefore makes it safe from the fear of consuming poisonous substances because nothing but heat is added. The dehydrated food will only maintain its initial nutrients and that makes it perfect for consumption.
7. Economic and Financial Advantages: Dehydrating food makes food last longer. As such, people may buy food in bulk or harvest large quantity of produce and dehydrate it in batches, making it a very convenient method.
8. Reliability for Emergency Situations: Dehydrating keeps a person prepared for any emergency that requires immediate need for dehydrated food. Dehydrated food can be very useful for individuals traveling in extreme conditions, such as for mountain climbers and cross-country bike riders.

DISADVANTAGES

1. Time Consumption: Dehydrating food requires a lot of time in order to achieve perfect results. Some foods have a large amount of water content and to reduce the water will require a lot of time and meticulous observation. Taking so much time may be inconvenient for some individuals.
2. Unwanted Weight Gain: Dehydrated food might be rich in calories. Since it has shrunken in size, it may appear small; a little quantity consumed may seems insufficient while a large quantity consumed implies large nutrient consumption. The excess calories in the dehydrated food may lead to weight gain. People should be aware of it when consuming dried food.
3. Loss of Nutrients: Although when done correctly, dehydrating food can preserve nutrients, when done incorrectly it may lead to loss of nutrients in the food. Some nutrients can't stand high levels of heat. The degree of heat applied therefore determines the survival of the nutrients in food. If the dehydrated food is not stored properly too, nutrient can be lost due to excessive heat and poor storage condition.
4. Change in Taste and Look: With high heat, the appetizing appearances of common meals change. In most cases, people are easily turned off when foods don't wear the expected looks. When foods are dehydrated, the loss of water makes it shrink and the looks drastically change.
5. Technical Knowledge: Since not all foods are dehydrated in the

same way or following the same pattern, dehydration requires technical knowledge in order to be carried out well. There is also the place of experience which gradually makes a person perfect in the art.

WHY IS DEHYDRATION HEALTHY?

Dehydration is healthy for consumption because of the following reasons:

1. Retains Nutrients: As mentioned earlier, when we dehydrate foods, the nutrients in the food is one of our primary concerns. Unlike other methods of preservation, dehydration saves the nutrients in the dehydrated food, when it is carried out effectively.
2. Bacteria Free: Dehydrated foods are germ-free. When we keep these foods for a long period of time, they still maintain their healthy state.
3. No Addition of External Chemicals: The heat used to dehydrate food is the only external requirement for the process. This heat contains no chemicals or acids that may be dangerous for the food. Unlike some preservative methods which engage the addition of preservative chemicals, dehydration is a healthy choice for storing food.
4. Safe Handling: Since dehydration has nothing to do with handling dangerous chemicals or intense equipment, it is safe for the user to easily dehydrate. Dehydration can be done with the simplest household mechanical devices like oven, microwave or a dehydrator. The smoke or steam that escapes from dehydrating food is not unhealthy to the environment, unlike regular burning of waste products. This makes the process healthy.

METHODS OF DEHYDRATION

Dehydration involves the following methods. Some of these are more industrial techniques and so won't be relevant for canning and preserving at home.

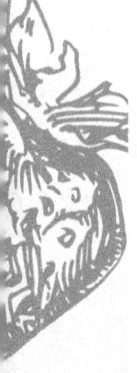

1. Drum Drying: Foods like fish and other small animals that requires whole rinsing are dehydrated with the aid of a drum dryer. Drum drying is used to dry out the liquids from raw materials to dehydrate them. It involves the use of low temperature in high capacity drums

with an overlaying metal sheet. The dehydrated foods are layered on the sheets and the water is gradually evaporated from the heat. In more recent times, drum drying retains the color and nutritional values of the dehydrated foods.

2. Microwave Vacuum Dryer: This is an electric microwave that provides heats to food by making electro-magnetic radiation available for it in the frequency range. Microwave vacuum dryers are oven-like and they make food heat up efficiently. These are commonly used in various kitchens and they are popular for warming previously cooked food, or cooking some simple foods like pop corns etc. These vacuum driers are also used in slowly applying heat to slow-heat requiring foods, which easily get burnt when cooked in pots and pans. Examples of foods cooked with these microwaves are margarines, hot butter, fats etc.

3. Iyophilisation or Cryodesiccation: This is also called 'Freeze Drying.' It is a dehydration process that requires low heat. It involves, first of all freezing the product and then gradually lowering the pressing, and finally getting rid of the ice through sublimation. The unique feature of this process is that unlike others which engage heat, this uses ice.

4. Spray Drying: This is the conversion of food materials to a dry powder. It involves the use of a drying product with a hot gas and converting them into liquid or slurry products. It is a common method of drying, acceptable for use in foods and pharmaceutical products. Spray driers use different atomizers or spray nozzles to disperse the liquid or slurry into a controlled drop sized spray.

5. Sun Drying: Sun drying is the earliest method of dehydration, and it is still in practice till date in some countries and deserts. It involves spreading food materials under the intense heat from the sun. Foods that are sundried usually maintain the tastes and can last effectively for a long period of time.

Sun drying is efficient for products like fish, meats and some solid dairy products. In some climes, sun dried products are half cooked and when ready for consumption, they are only further partially cooked and consumed. Sun drying can greatly improve the taste of the food while it makes it more nourishing.

Advantages of Sun Drying

1. Sun drying involves no equipment or fire. It makes use of natural sunlight for drying.
2. It saves energy and costs, and makes food last longer.
3. It improves the taste and nutrients of food.

Disadvantages of Sun Drying

1. In some areas, fleas and insects can perch on the food when open to the environment.
2. If not properly done, the heating process may not be intense and the food may not be well dehydrated.

Chapter 6.
Smoking

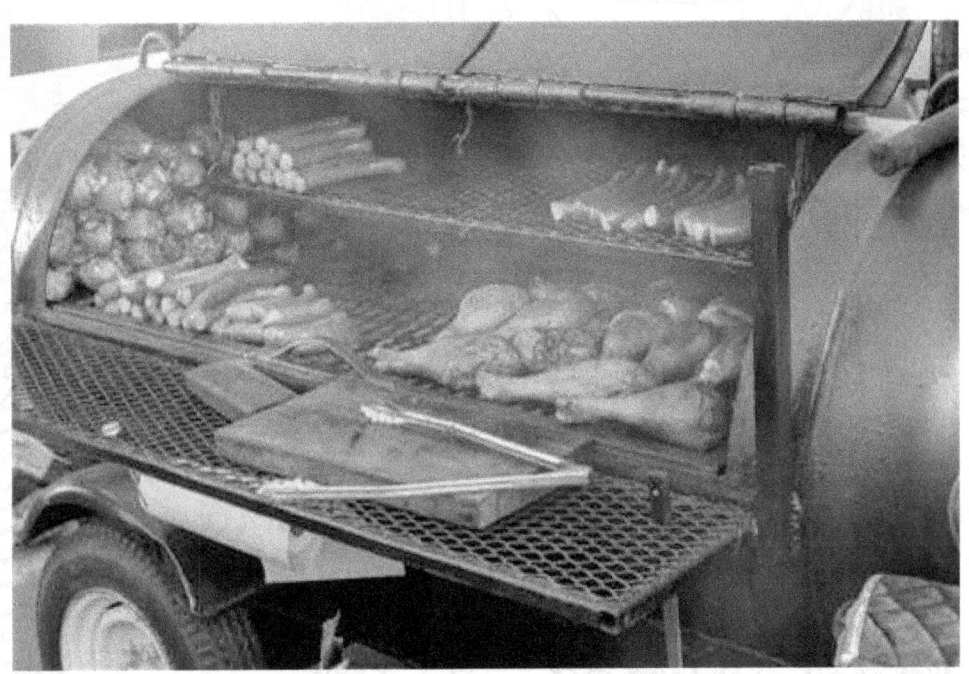

Many people may discount smoking food, particularly meat, as an effective method of food preservation since smoking meat is the most renowned as the best way to flavor meat with smoke (hence the term, 'smoking meat'). In reality, smoking meat is also an effective way of food preservation that has been used for centuries. In today's modern world though, we often smoke our meat with smoke houses that are made of sanitary, safe materials. Indeed, meat smoking does enhance the taste of the meat, but it all depends on the time and density of the smoking process. There are many great methods for smoking meat, as well as many benefits to it. When you smoke meat, it can either come out really good, or really bad.

Smoking meat delivers many improvements for the meat that goes beyond the taste and texture of it. This is where the food preservation part comes in. Smoking means that it will preserve the meat by drastically slowing down the spread of the growth of bacteria. The part of the meat that will almost always spoil the fastest is the fat. Smoking is effective because it increases the amount of time it will take for the fat of the meat to spoil. As a result, the overall shelf life of the meat is dramatically increased. Smoking meat also leads to water loss, which will lead to a naturally increased shelf life, as the meat itself will be both drier and saltier.

The smell and changed color of smoked meat can be overpowering. Meat can change to a red, brown or black color, and smoked fish will turn golden. The best way to properly smoke meat is to do so at your home, since most smoked meat products at grocery stores and supermarkets are not properly smoked and will lack a prolonged shelf life. For example, a properly smoked sausage will take a good part of three days to properly smoke, to really increase the shelf life and the taste and color of it, but very few manufacturers will take the time and effort to do that. Instead, manufacturers use 'special' chemicals and liquid smoke to smoke the meat. This also keeps the overall price of the meats down and increases profits for the manufacturer and/or retailer. These manufacturers assume that you will put the meat in a refrigerator or freezer first anyway, which alone will drastically decrease the overall flavor and color of the meat.

Plain and simple, the overwhelming majority of store bought smoked meats are not truly smoked meats, in terms of both, taste and shelf life/preservation. The best way to smoke meat is to buy some regular meat and then smoke it at your home. The question then is, how can you properly smoke meat at your home to make it both taste good and increase its shelf life?

The most common types of smoked meats are pork. This includes bacon, ribs, loins, roasts, back fat, hams, and smaller piece of meat. Most pieces of meat are large sized, requiring large smoking and cooking times to completely cure the meat of harmful microorganisms and bacteria, and to increase the shelf life of it. There are many other methods for preparing these meats as well, such as barbecuing, cooking in the oven, boiling, frying, etc. But smoking the meat will almost always result in the best combination of both taste and preservation.

There are two steps that must be followed when smoking meat. The first step is to, well, smoke it in the smokehouse. This alone will cure the harmful bacteria and microorganisms in the meat. The next step is optional, but it is to cook it, and it can either increase or decrease the quality of your meat depending on how you cook it. When you cook the meat afterwards, you control the temperature; have a reliable supply of heat, and excellent insulation to maintain those levels of heat and temperature if the weather is poor outside.

You should cook your meat at approximately 170 degrees Fahrenheit after it has been smoked. The overall quality of your meat will largely depend on having the correct temperature, especially since the actual smoking process is performed well less than 170 degrees Fahrenheit. As for the actual smoking process, the meat should be smoked at less than 160 degrees Fahrenheit. This way, you will avoid the danger of food poisoning, toxins, and exhibit a traditional color of smoked meat. You can also smoke your meats without the use of nitrates, but to do this you will need to smoke the meat at a higher temperature than the normal cooking heat of 170 degrees Fahrenheit. You also increase the risks of not eliminating all the bacteria and microorganisms that are harmful to the meat, because nitrates are a cure for those harmful substances. However, it can still be done without the use of nitrates; it just needs to be smoked at an increased temperature. In addition, smoking without nitrates would best be done in a self-contained smoker, where the air that is incoming from the outside is kept to a minimum. This reduces the chance of the smoke bursting into flames.

A large smokehouse, especially one that is completely inside, will have a much greater chance of having fresh air flow into it from the outside. If you do have a large, outdoor smokehouse, using dry wood will increase safety since less moisture is created.

It can truly not be enunciated enough that the temperature of smoking and cooking meat is extremely important. Another reason why manufactured smoked meat is typically at a lower level of quality is because manufacturers do not smoke it at proper levels. This tip may also be confusing since another rule is that there is no decisive temperature that will decide the quality of your meat. This is because all meat is different, but you might be comforted in knowing that a difference of just a few degrees from where your meat should be smoked at, will not lead to a large decrease in quality. A good bar to set for yourself is to never increase the inside temperature of the smokehouse to be greater than 170 degrees Fahrenheit, as the fat of the meat will melt quickly, and once the fat is melted, the inside of the meat will be a mess, and lack taste and extended shelf life.

It's also important that when you plan on smoking meat, the meat you buy or prepare beforehand, is of good quality. If your meat is greasy on the outside or inside, is shriveled, is dense and thick, looks or smells old, or falls apart too easily, then you should avoid smoking that meat (and perhaps avoid eating it entirely!)

This is why smoking temperatures are so important, because even if you smoke meat that is of good quality beforehand, a drastic increase or decrease in temperature from what it should be at could change the quality of your meat to the quality that you wouldn't have bought beforehand.

It's also important to know the amount of smoke that you are smoking your meat at. When making your decision about how much smoke to use, hopefully these factors will influence your decision: typically, the thicker the smoke is, the faster your meat will smoke, and high levels of humidity in your smokehouse will lead to a less flavorful color of your meat. This is also true to the surface of your meat itself; if it is moist, this will also lead to less colorful meat. In addition, a higher temperature in the smokehouse will also lead to a faster smoking process, and it's important that you get at least some smoke from the outside to the inside of your smokehouse. It's just important that you don't get too much inside, since a fast enough air speed will cause damage to your meat.

The final question regarding the smoking of meat is how long you should smoke it. Just as with the amount of smoke or the temperature that you should smoke your meat at, there is no decisive time as to how long you should smoke your meat, as all meat is different. If you want to remove the moisture of your meat, however, then you can use cold smoking methods, which will take very long days or even weeks to be successful. Unfortunately, many people lack the patience to smoke meat for this long. Another alternative is hot smoking, which leads to much shorter times, and also will lead to the overall best flavor of the meat. Sometimes, hot smoking will only require a time period of just a few hours. This is especially true for sausages, which have a small diameter and therefore require much less time to properly smoke.

Chapter 7.
Canning and Preserving Tools

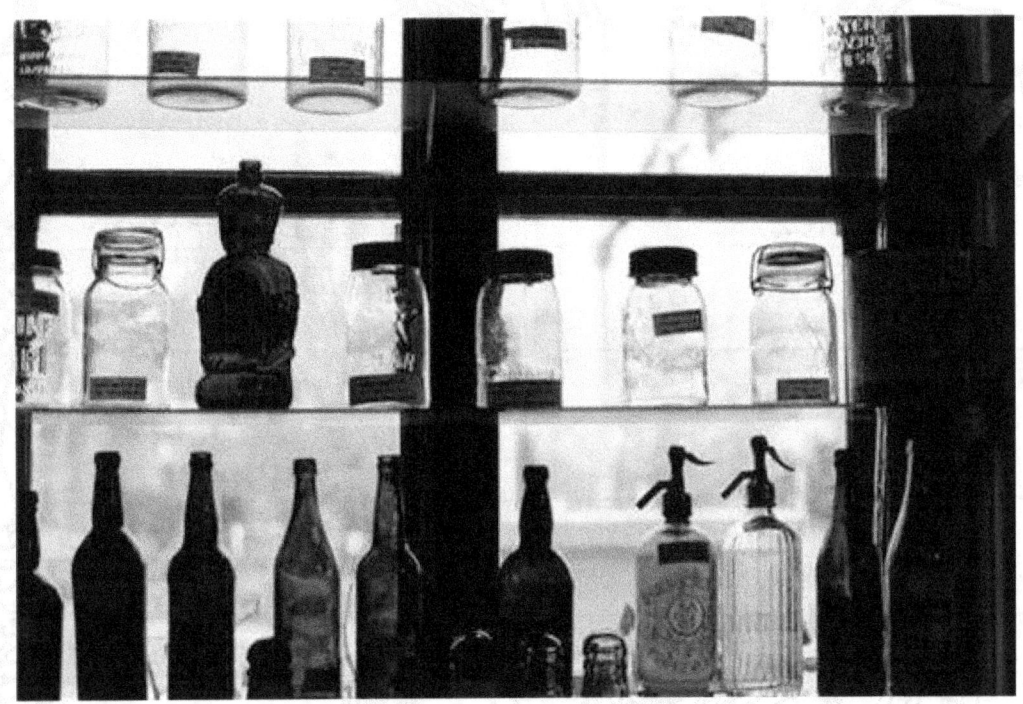

CANNING JARS

Not all jars were made for canning. When we talk about canning jars, they are available in various sizes and finishes. It all depends on what you are planning to can. Here is the info to guide you in selecting the right jars:

- *Quart Jars:* You can use these jars for large foods, for example, whole tomatoes or for a generous amount, such as soup for many people or spaghetti sauce. These jars are available in regular-mouth and wide-mouth styles.

- *Pint Jars:* This is the most versatile-size jar; the container can hold just about anything: veggies to serve one or two people, relishes, pickles, and smaller amounts of sauces. Pint jars are available in regular-mouth and wide-mouth style.

- Half-Pint Jars: These jars spot straight interior sides that allow you to get every last bit out of each jar. Regular-mouth jars are taller than broad-mouth half-pint jars. Some have a quilt or other design on the exterior.

- 4-Ounce Jars: These are small jars that can contain amounts you intend to can in small portions, or will quickly use. They are great choices of jars if you are making a big batch of jam for your family and friends.

Jars (oz.)	Types of Food
4	Jams, Jellies, Mustard, Sauces, Ketchup, Flavored Vinegar
8	Jams, Jellies, Fruit Preserve, Fruit Syrup, Pizza Sauce, Chutney
12	Jams, Jellies, Marmalade
16	Sauces, Salsa, Relish, Pie Filling
32	Fruits, Vegetables, Meats

- Decorative Jars: These glass jars are perfect for refrigerator-pickled foods that do not call for heat processing. Just ensure to clean them in hot, soapy water and rinse properly prior to filling them.

- Vintage Jars: These are old canning jars with spring-type lids or colored glass. Though they're pretty collector pieces, they should not be used in modern canning. They do not seal properly, may crack, and have uneven sizes. Do not use them for canning; rather, display them on a shelf.

- Make sure you use only standard canning jars. They're made to resist the heat in a canner, and their mouths are especially threaded to be properly sealed with canning lids. You won't be happy to find your canned food spoiled soon after. Examine them carefully before using and get rid of any chipped or cracked ones.

To take out hard-water film or mineral deposits, soak unfilled jars in a solution of one cup of vinegar per gallon of water. Purchase canning jars in grocery, in discount, or in hardware stores, or order them online.

- *Wide-Mouth and Regular-Mouth Canning Jars:* Wide-mouth canning jars make packing whole vegetables and fruits into a jar easier. They are suitable for foods like pickles since the broad mouth makes it easier to use your fingers or utensils to take out just a pickle at a time.

- *Regular-mouth canning jars are the pints and quart jars that have shoulders. Wide mouth half-pint jars are shorter than the regular-mouth ones. The latter mouths are narrower than the former, and they are perfect for soups, sauces, or crushed vegetables and fruits.*

- *Screw Bands and Canning Lids:* Make sure you follow the maker's directions when you are making use of screw bands and canning lids. The former is crucial for locking the latter to the jars during processing. You may remove the bands after processing, if you want, as they are technically no longer required; the screw bands offer some cushioning between jars when placed on shelves. You can only reuse screw bands if they are not rusty or bent. Purchase bands and lids in grocery, in discount, or in hardware stores, although they are often sold with their corresponding canning jars.

Canning lids are made for a one-time use and its best to purchase them for the current canning season. When stored, some sealing composites lose efficacy, so the ideal thing is purchasing new lids right before canning. Lids are sized to fit the wide mouth and regular mouth jars. If buying new jars, bands and lids would be incorporated, but you can buy lids separately as well. You only need to make sure you are buying the right size for your jars. The colored substance underneath the lid is the sealing composite that helps seal the lid onto the jar.

- *Water-Bath or Boiling-Water Canner:* A water-bath canner heats the jar to 212 degrees F, which is sufficient to get rid of microbes found in high-acid foods. The rack enables the flow of water underneath the jars for smooth heating and has handles that enable you to easily lower and raise jars into the warm water. There are different sizes and forms of canners. A conventional freckled enameled model might rust and chip over time; if you intend to make canning a leisure pursuit, high-end boiling-water canners are also available in glossy polished steel.

If it is available, a large stock-pot with a tight-fitting lid that will contain many jars that are a few inches deeper than their height can be used as a canner. A rack will still be useful to set up jars from the base of the pot to enable smooth flow of water beneath them and evenly heat the jars. If you don't want to do a lot of canning, this can be a great solution.

Make use of a water bath canner for tomatoes, fruits (if you add lemon juice or other acidic ingredients), marmalades, jams, relishes, jellies, and pickles. Since these foods contain a higher acidity than vegetables, you do not need to use a pressure canner to process them. Pressure Canner: Would you like to can some extra vegetables in the garden? The only tool you need is a pressure canner! This type of canner is what you will use for low-acid foods like vegetables. It will come with a heavy pot that has a rack, a tight-fitting lid with a petcock or vent, a safety fuse, and a weighted or dial pressure gauge.

These types of canners enable you to heat foods to 240 or 250 degrees F, and that temperature can be maintained for as long as required. There are different types of pressure canners with different features, so always check the directions of the manufacturer before you begin to use one. Purchase your pressure canners from anyplace where they sell cooking equipment.

CANNING-SPECIFIC TOOLS

Besides your canner and your jars, there are a few other pieces of equipment that are especially important for canning. You will normally find special kits to purchase that will have all of the necessary extra tools such as a magnetic lid wand, a funnel, and a jar lifter (this will save you time from searching out all the materials separately). Make sure you wash (with soap and warm water) any tools that will have contact with the food prior to using them.

- *Jar Funnels:* Do not use just any funnel for canning! Jar funnels are much shorter and wider than other funnels, they are available in both regular-mouth and wide-mouth versions. They are very helpful for preventing spills in the course of filling jars, they also make guiding your food inside the canning jars easier (especially sauces or crushed vegetables and fruits).

- *Jar-Lifter:* This utensil raises jars in and out of warm water tightly and securely. Use both your hands and tightly squeeze. Kitchen tongs can also be used, but they aren't as secure. This essential tool is not only meant for lifting your jars of veggies in and out of the canner, but it is also useful when sterilizing the jars before you begin.

- *Combination Ruler/Spatula:* A canning spatula will help you to get the most out of every jar. This utensil's notched end is designed to match the most common jars' headspace. It is a bit flexible with a tapered end, making it the perfect device for slipping in to release air bubbles along the sides of filled jars.

- *Magnetic Lid Wand:* This wand makes it easier for you to drop rings and lids into the canner's warm water to sterilize them, makes the sealing composite softer, and quickly raises and takes them out. When you have this device, there is no need for heating lids in a separate pot. It makes attaching the lid to each jar a bit straightforward, and thus saves you time.

IMPORTANT TIPS:

- Always follow the instructions precisely, use the recommended pressure and time for processing foods.
- To arrive at the correct processing time, start timing once the requisite pressure is attained in a pressure canner, or once the water has returned to boiling inside a boiling water canner.
- Bear in mind food safety, as mentioned in Chapter 1! Always check each of the home-canned jars cautiously before serving. If you observe a leaking jar, a swollen lid, or patches of mold or that the food has a murky or foamy look, dispose of the jar with the food.
- When you open a jar, the smell from it ought to be pleasant. If the food does not smell or look nice, do not use it.
- As an additional safeguard, cook pressure-canned veggies for

nothing less than ten minutes before serving.

OTHER ITEMS NEEDED

All of these tools may not be required when you are canning, but surely they can be helpful. The following are some additional tools you may need to have at your disposal:

- *Kitchen scale*
- *Vegetable peeler, a sharp knife, and a cutting board*
- *Dutch oven or large kettle and saucepan*
- *Cheesecloth, a jelly bag, colander, a food mill, a sieve*
- *Large spoon or ladle and wide-mouth funnel*
- *Wooden spoon, plastic knife, or rubber scraper*
- *Paper towels or clean clothes*
- *Magnetic-tip lid wand, jar lifter, ruler*
- *Wire rack, hot pads, and a kitchen timer*

Chapter 8.
Canning and Preserving Tips

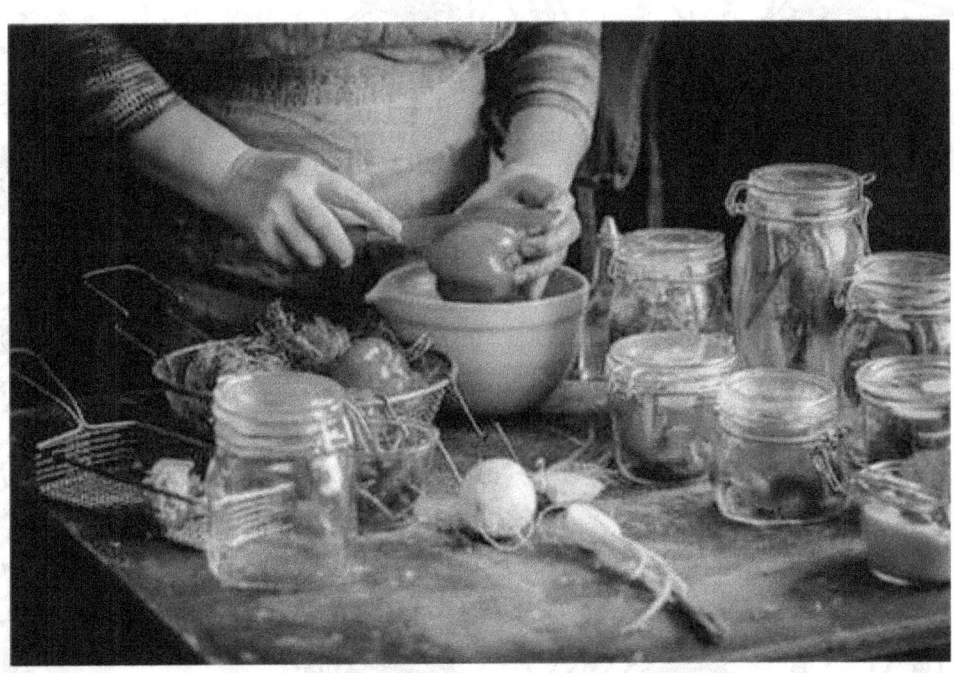

There are a few safety tips that you should follow when you start canning and preserving foods from home. Canning is a great way to store and preserve foods, but it can be risky if not done correctly. However, if you follow these tips, you will be able to can foods in a safe manner.

CHOOSE THE RIGHT CANNER

The first step to safe home canning is choosing the right canner. First off, know when to use a pressure canner or a water bath canner. Use a pressure canner that is specifically designed for canning and preserving foods. There are several types of canners out there and some are just for cooking food, not for preserving food and processing jars. Be sure that you have the right type of equipment. Make sure your pressure canner is the right size. If your canner is too small, the jars may be undercooked. Always opt for a larger canner as the pressure on the bigger pots tends to be more accurate, and you will be able to take advantage of the larger size and can more foods at once!

Before you begin canning, check that your pressure canner is in good condition. If your canner has a rubber gasket, it should be flexible and soft. If the rubber is dry or cracked, it should be replaced before you start canning. Be sure your canner is clean and the small vents in the lid are free of debris. Adjust your canner for high altitude processing if needed.

Once you are sure your canner is ready to go and meets all these guidelines, it is time to start canning!

OPT FOR A SCREW TOP LID SYSTEM

There are many kinds of canning jars that you can choose to purchase. However, the only type of jar that is approved by the USDA is a mason jar with a screw-top lid. These are designated 'preserving jars,' and are considered the safest and most effective option for home preserving uses.

Some jars are not thought to be safe for home preservation despite being marketed as canning jars. Bail Jars, for example, have a two-part wire clasp lid, with a rubber ring in between the lid and jar. While these were popular in the past, it is now thought that the thick rubber and tightly closed lid does not provide a sufficient seal, leading to a higher potential for botulism. Lightening Jars should not be used for canning as they are simply glass jars with glass lids, with no rubber at all. That will not create a good seal!

Reusing jars from store-bought products is another poor idea. They may look like they're in good condition, but they are typically designed to be processed in a commercial facility. Most store-bought products do not have the two-part band and lid system, which is best for home canning. Also, the rubber seal on a store-bought product is likely not reusable once you open the original jar. You can reuse store-bought jars at home for storage, but not for canning and preserving.

CHECK YOUR JARS, LIDS, AND BANDS

As you wash your jars with soapy water, check for any imperfections. Even new jars may have a small chip or crack and need to be discarded. You can reuse jars again and again, as long as they are in good condition.

The metal jar rings are also reusable; however, you should only reuse them if they are rust free and undented. If your bands begin to show signs of wear, consider investing in some new ones.

Jar lids need to be new as the sealing compound on the lid can disintegrate over time. When you store your jars in damp places (like in a basement or canning cellar) the lids are even more likely to disintegrate. Always use new lids to ensure that your canning is successful.

CHECK FOR RECENT CANNING UPDATES

Canning equipment has changed over the years, becoming more high tech and therefore more efficient at processing foods. In addition to the equipment becoming more advanced, there have also been many scientific improvements, making canning safer when the proper steps are taken. For example, many people used to sterilize their jars before pressure canning.

Make sure that your food preservation information is all up to date and uses current canning guidelines. Avoid outdated cookbooks and reassess 'trusted family methods' to make sure they fit into the most recent criteria for safe canning. When in doubt, check with the 'US Department of Agriculture's Complete Guide to Home Canning,' which contains the most recent, up-to-date canning tips.

PICK THE BEST INGREDIENTS

When choosing food to can, always get the best food possible. You want to use high quality, perfectly ripe produce for canning. You will never end up with a jar of food better than the product itself, so picking good ingredients is important to the taste of your final product. Also, products that past its prime can affect the ability to can it. If strawberries are overripe, your jam may come out too runny. If your tomatoes are past their prime, they may not have a high enough pH level to be processed in a water bath. Pick your ingredients well and *you will make successful preserved foods.*

CLEAN EVERYTHING

While you may know that your jars and lids need to be washed and sanitized, don't forget about the rest of your tools. Cleaning out your canner before using it is essential, even if you put it away clean. Make sure to wipe your countertop well, making sure there are no crumbs or residue. Wash your produce with clean, cold water and don't forget to wash your hands! The cleaner everything is, the less likely you are to spread bacteria onto your jarred foods

FOLLOW YOUR RECIPE

Use recipes from trusted sources and be sure to follow them to the letter. Changing the amount of one or two ingredients may alter the balance of acidity and could result in unsafe canning (especially when using a water bath canner). Use the ingredients as directed and make very few changes, none if possible.

Adhere to the processing times specified by your recipe. Sometimes the times may seem a little long, but the long processing time is what makes these products safe to store on the shelf. The processing time is the correct amount of time needed to destroy spoilage organisms, mold spores, yeast and pathogens in the jar. So, as you may have guessed, it is extremely important to use the times that are written in your recipe as a hard rule.

COOL THE JARS

Be sure that you give your jars 12 hours to cool before testing the seal. If you test the seal too early, it may break as the jar is still warm, making the rubber pliable. Be sure to cool the jars away from a window or fan, as even a slight breeze may cause the hot jars to crack. Once cool, remove the metal band, clean it and save it for your next canning project.

DON'T RISK IT

If you suspect that the food you have canned is bad, don't try to eat it, just toss it! Each time you open a jar of canned food, inspect it and check for the following:

1. Is the lid bulging, swollen, or leaking at all?
2. If the jar is cracked or damaged?
3. Does the jar foam when opened?
4. Is the food inside discolored or moldy?
5. Does the food smell bad?

If you notice any of these warning signs in a food that you have canned, throw it away. Do not taste it to check if it is good. It is not worth risking your health to try the food after seeing one of the above signs.
Avoid using overripe fruit, as canning is not designed to improve the food's quality. If quality is low at the start of the process, it will worsen in storage.

Do not put more ingredients with low acid (garlic, celery, onions and pepper) than what the recipe specifies. This can make the product unsafe.

Do not add a significant amount of spices or seasoning than what is recommended as these items usually have high bacteria levels, and too much spices is able to make the item unsafe.

Avoid the use of fat or butter for home canning unless it is suggested in a trial recipe. These ingredients are not good for storing and can increase the spoilage rate. When fat or butter is added, this can also slow down the heat transfer rate and renders the product unsafe.

For thickeners, do not use flour, starches or add barley, pasta or rice to the canned products. This goes for pickled items and sauces, and also savory products such as stews and soups. 'Clear-Jel' can be added as this was tested in food labs in universities and also in USDA. Items used to thicken products absorb liquid in the process and causes the way the food heats to slow down. This may end up in under-processing and the food being unsafe.

Acid such as vinegar, citric acid or lemon should be added to any product with tomato.

Food scientists in 1994 found the danger of botulism poisoning derived from tomato canned products and there is now the recommendation for acid to be added to tomatoes that are canned, and even to the ones canned commercially. Lemon juice can be found everywhere but will give the canned tomatoes a sharp taste; the flavor will be less noticeably changed with citric acid, and a lot of recipes have vinegar included.

Jars should never be processed in an oven such as microwave, gas or electric. Steam canning also is not generally recommended. There will be some manufacturers that market steam canners, but it will be found that there are practically no credible establishments that recommend them. This is for various reasons, which begins with basic properties of heat transfers of steam versus water.

PREVENTING DARKENING

Some cut or peeled fruits like apples, nectarines and peaches will become dark when they are left open to air. Darkening can be prevented with any of the simple techniques listed below:

- Use commercial ascorbic mixture of acid such as 'Fruit-Fresh,' and sprinkle it over cut fruit. Mix it well. This can be found at any drug and grocery stores.
- Place cut fruit in a solution of ascorbic acid (1 teaspoon) and a gallon of water. This vitamin C is available at drug stores in powered form. Allow it to drain before canning.
- Put cut fruit in solution of lemon juice; ¾ cup of lemon juice to a gallon of water. Fruit should be drained before canning.

CANNING JARS

For home canning, use regular jars like mason, Kerr, Ball etc. The food jars that are commercially used, like mayonnaise jars, are not tempered by heat and frequently break easily. Spaghetti jars of brands like 'Classico' are known to be ideal for this purpose, also. Sealing can also be difficult if the sealing surfaces are not exactly fitting the canning lids. Ensure that every closure and jar is perfect. Throw out any that are dented, chipped, rusty or cracked. Airtight seals will be prevented if there are any defects.

Only the jar size that is specified in the recipe should be used, because the product may become unsafe. Most times a smaller size can be used. In general, the largest size to be used is a quartz size.

Hard water films and scales can be removed from jars by soaking them in a vinegar solution (1 cup to 1 gallon of water). Jars must be kept warm until it is time to fill them. This cut down on breakage is caused by thermal shock.

Flat lids may be used only one time, but while screw bands remain in good condition, they can be reused. The lids from foods that are commercially canned should not be reused at all.

ADDITIONAL TIPS ON WATER BATH CANNING

- Put water halfway in the canner.
- When required, preheat the water to be added to the jar to a temperature that is very warm, yet, not boiling, about (140°F), for foods that are raw-packed; low temperatures assist in reducing jar breakage; boiling water should be used for the hot-packed foods.
- Continue to add boiling water if required to ensure that the water level is a minimum of one inch over the jar tops.
- Cover the canner, and if required, lower the heat settings for maintaining a gentle but full boil, for the duration of the process time. It is recommended that the heat remains on high.
- Two burners can be used at one time if a single burner is not enough to produce the required heat.
- Retightening of the jar lids can break its seal.
- Ensure that the jars are not left in boiling water when the processing time is completed as food will be overcooked.
- Inspect jar seals for breaks and leaks within 12 to 24 hours after they are processed. Press on the lid and if it is sealed, it will be tightly pulled down. If it is not sealed, it will give off a kind of exploding sound with each tip.
- For storing, take off screw bands, then wipe jars clean. If this is not done, the rings might rust and securely attach to the jar.

Luckily, it is fairly easy to spot a jar of food that has gone bad. Home-canned food can spoil for many reasons. A dent in the lid, a small crack in the jar, an improper seal, or not enough processing time are all common errors that may cause canned foods to go bad. Follow the exact canning directions and hopefully, you will never get a bad jar of food!

UNSAFE CANNING METHODS

The general consensus is that the only two safe methods of canning are the two described in this book: Pressure Canning and Boiling Water Canning.

A number of other canning methods have been handed down from generation to generation. If you're using a method other than the two described in this book, you're endangering yourself and your family.

I hear people say all the time, "It hasn't made me sick yet and we've been doing it for years."

Remember this bit of wisdom: Just because it hasn't made you sick yet, doesn't mean it can't make you sick. Other methods of canning can make you sick or even kill you. Botulism isn't something you want to play around with. Its undetectable using your sense of smell, sight or taste and the effects can be deadly.

Here are some of the methods known to be unsafe:

- Oven Canning: The heat an oven gives off is unreliable at best. Temperatures may not be what you think they are and jars heated in an oven tend to heat unevenly.
- Dishwasher Canning: It's OK to use your dishwasher to sterilize jars prior to using them for canning. It's NOT OK to use it during the actual canning process.
- Aspirin Canning: This is an old method used many, many years ago. Aspirin is added to food before it's put in canning jars. This is one of the most dangerous methods of canning, as the aspirin does absolutely nothing to preserve the food.
- Open-Kettle Canning: The food is cooked and put into hot jars, but the jars aren't boiled or pressurized to ensure a good seal. This method doesn't sufficiently process the foods being canned. It also allows air to be trapped in the jars, which promotes decomposition.
- Wax Canning: Wax is used to seal the jars. This method doesn't provide a good seal and fails to properly process the food.

Chapter 9.
Benefits of Canning and Preserving

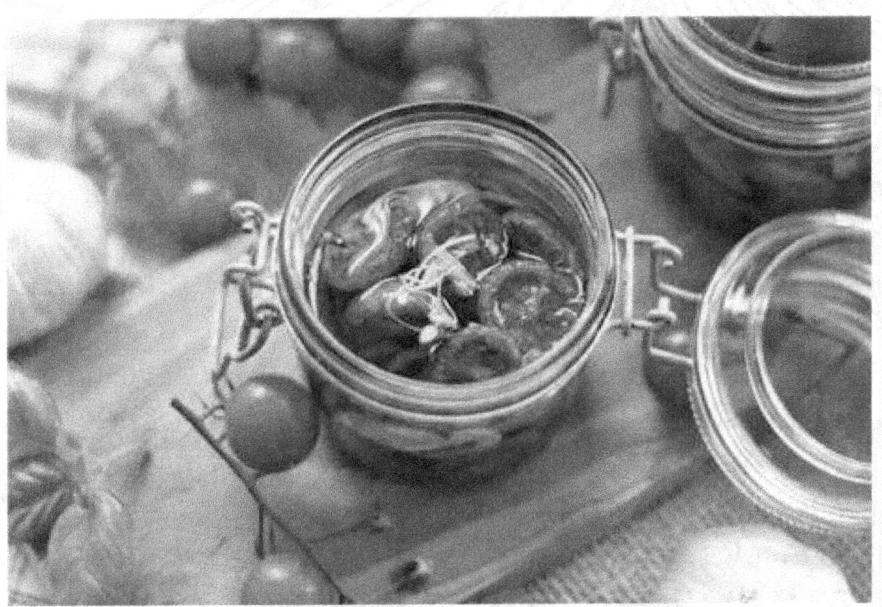

NUTRITION

Fresh produce, like fruits and vegetables, are known to start 'dying' and lose their vitamins from the moment they are harvested from the ground. Up to half, or even more of the vitamins may be lost within a few days if the fruits or vegetables are not stored in a cool place or preserved appropriately. It takes up to two weeks for refrigerated produce to lose its vitamins and start deteriorating. If fresh produce is harvested, cleaned, and stored in a good time, the majority of its vitamins will be preserved. Fruits and vegetables that are harvested and canned properly will be able to be of higher nutritional value than fresh produce that is stored in makeshift conditions.

The problem with a lot of products that is sold in commercial facilities these days is that a number of chemicals and substances have been used to improve the appearance of the produce, and its shelf life too. Fresh produce, when exposed for a long amount of time, will become home to microorganisms, regardless of the storage conditions. Some shops are neglectful with their products and this ends up affecting the health of consumers. When you choose to can your own food and even grow your own produce, you can avoid using potentially harmful substances. Canning is simply preserving fresh food in its original state. The preservatives that you will use are also natural; acids such as lemon juice or vinegar are known to have a great number of benefits for the human body.

ECONOMICAL

As mentioned above, fresh produce is not able to last for long; it isn't cheap, either. Canning can be very useful for a person, especially when it comes to preserving seasonal fruits and vegetables. The price of seasonal produce is usually high and after a certain amount of time, it becomes hard to find these fruits and vegetables again. Canning allows you to preserve fruits, vegetables (and other foods) in bulk, allowing you to keep a steady supply of vegetables for a longer period of time, and for a lesser amount of money. If you are into planting and harvesting your own produce, this will slash your food expenses in half. You will be able to rule out buying produce regularly since you'll be supplying yourself with your own stock. If you have business acumen, you could look into starting a small business of your own. If not, that's okay. At least you will have a ready supply of fruits and vegetables at any time you want. If you are a fan of homemade jams that they sell in stores, you will be pleased to know that you will be able to make your own, with your own canned fruits and vegetables, and at a lower cost. Canning really is a much more economical option in comparison to buying produce on a daily/weekly basis.

DURABILITY

Cans are able to withstand extreme conditions: heat, cold, wet, dry, etc. This means you can store your canned food in almost any kind of environment without worrying about the condition of the can. What you do need to watch out for, though, are signs of rusting, leakage, denting or bulging; these are signs that could mean that the cans have been damaged and the food has been affected.

INCREASED SHELF LIFE

The process of canning, which involves the use of high temperatures and very sterile containers, ensures that any organism that can cause spoilage is destroyed. As long as the container remains intact, the food will remain safe. Once a container is compromised, you have to throw the food out in order to avoid anyone from contracting harmful diseases or infections. Canning is able to provide a shelf life that can span anywhere from one to four or five years. The shelf life can be longer than this under certain circumstances; some products are known to have a shelf life of over thirty years.

In 1974, samples of canned food from an 1865 wreck of a steamboat, Bertrand, were processed and analyzed by the National Food Processors Association; the results were astounding. Despite the deterioration of the food's appearance, odor, and vitamin content the food was otherwise preserved and healthy to eat!

You won't need your food to last for over one hundred years, but it will definitely last longer than a couple of months. Canning is an effective method for families to incorporate into their lifestyles because it saves mothers and fathers from spending money every day on the produce for daily meals. If you are someone who personally grows and harvests your own produce, canning will be a great way for you to preserve your harvest. Having a long shelf life means you can create a food supply without worrying about the food spoiling or rotting in a short space of time.

REWARDING EXPERIENCE

Canning your own food is also a very rewarding personal experience. It can easily become a skill or hobby you develop for your spare time. Canning involves mental and physical work, which improves your body in more ways than one. It can also be a good experience for couples and families since it is something that can be done as a group. You will get to educate your children on the origins of the food that they eat, and you will also be teaching them a very useful skill that could be passed down in your family. If you are a sucker for old school, canning is also a great thing for you as it will rouse nostalgia within you. Many canners have spoken of the sentimental connection they have developed with canning, because it reminds them of earlier times in their childhood.

IT'S ECO-FRIENDLY TOO

The problem with the produce that is sold in commercial facilities is that the process of preserving them is not environmentally friendly. The facilities that are used to cool produce run on electricity, which is generated by fossil fuels. We all already know how bad the burning of fossil fuels is for the environment. Produce is also stored in plastic containers which are discarded off after the produce has been consumed. Plastic materials are never good for the environment because they are not biodegradable.

Chapter 10.
Vegetable Recipes

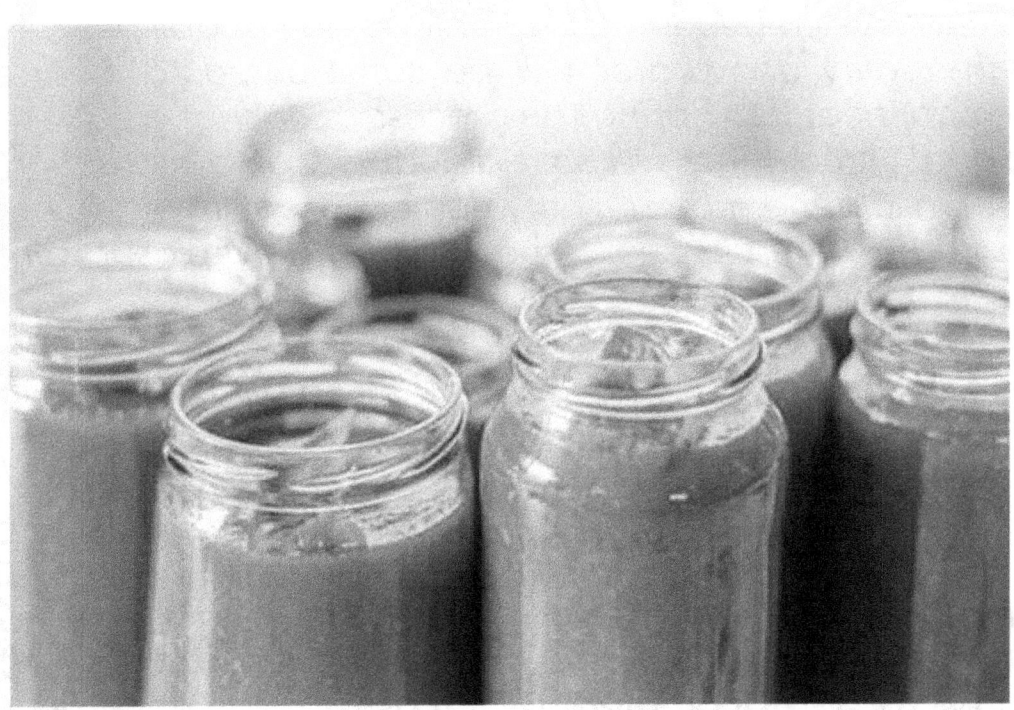

DEHYDRATING FRUITS AND VEGETABLES

There are four separate methods that allow you to dry fruits and vegetables. Each has both positives and negatives, and I will outline them:

FOOD DEHYDRATOR

The majority of people who dehydrate their fruits and vegetables use an electric dehydrator. There are many reasons.

1. They are consistent and produce a quality product.
2. They are of high quality and reasonably priced.
3. They do not require a lot of care and are very simple to use.

4. They provide flexibility, unlike other methods.

There are requirements that your food dehydrator should have:

1. It should have a thermostatically regulated temperature dial. It should have settings between 130 °F and 150 °F.
2. It will need to have a fan or blower to make sure that the warm air is evenly distributed.
3. It should have shelves that are made of stainless steel and a good grade of plastic.
4. It should have easy loading and unloading capabilities.
5. A high-quality dehydrator will be constructed to minimize the amount of heat loss during the process of drying.
6. High quality machines will have a double-wall construction, with a layer of insulating material between each wall to retain heat.
7. The external cabinets should be made of hard plastic, aluminum or steel.
8. It should have an enclosed heating element.
9. It should offer a selection of tray options (most have between 4 to 10 food trays).
10. Ensure that spare parts are readily available and these parts should be reasonably priced.

SUN DRYING FRUITS AND VEGETABLES

There are lot of factors that come into consideration when you are using the sun to dry your food.

1. The temperature outside needs to be above 90 °F.
2. The humidity must be low.
3. Air pollution must be low.
4. You will need to purchase drying trays and a protective netting to prevent bugs from bothering your food.

Unfortunately, there are many disadvantages to drying your food using a sun drying method.

1. You are exclusively dependent on temperature, humidity and air quality.
2. If the climate changes from one day to the next, you will need to

use a backup method to complete the process. If you do not have a backup method, your food will spoil.
3. In cooler nights, the food must be moved indoors.
4. It can take 2 to 4 days to dry foods using the sun, compared to 6 to 8 hours using an electric food dehydrator.

SOLAR DRYING

Solar dryers use the heat of the sun but at a more intense level. This method gives you a higher drying temperature, which means that your food dries faster. The faster the food dries, the quicker the microorganisms and enzymes on food will die faster.
Solar drying works by using a box that collects the sun's rays; this increases the temperature you get the affect mentioned above.
You can build your own solar dryer using various methods that are easily found online.
You have the ability to enclose your food from all sides.

OVEN DRYING METHODS

There are many advantages of using a regular oven:

1. Not dependent on weather
2. Regulated heat
3. Very little to no investment

There are more disadvantages of using an oven dyer than there are positives.

1. Drying fruits and vegetables in the oven will provide you with safe and tasty food. However, it does not provide the high quality that you would get from a dehydrator.
2. Energy costs are significant if you are drying a large quantity of fruits and vegetables.
3. The oven must be capable of maintaining a steady temperature. You do not want the food to cook, you want it to dehydrate.
4. Using your oven for a sustained period of time to dehydrate food prevents you from using it for other purposes.

If you decide to use the oven:

1. *You will need to test the oven's ability to maintain a steady temperature.*
2. *The oven door must be left open when testing or drying fruit.*
3. *Using your oven thermometer to test the oven for 1 hour prior to drying, you must make sure that it maintains a temperature between 130 °F and 150 °F.*
4. *Temperatures on either side of the range will either cook instead of drying, or cause the food to spoil.*

1. Asparagus, Spears

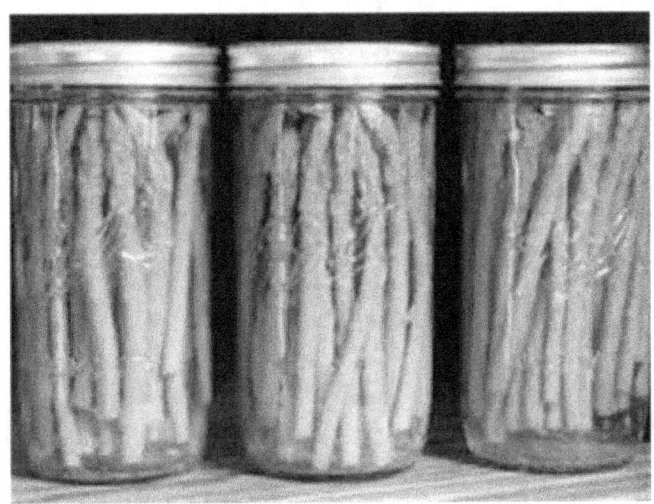

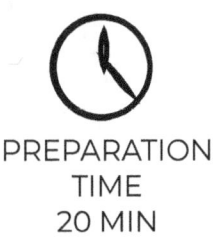

PREPARATION TIME
20 MIN

COOK TIME
30 MIN

SERVING
9 PINTS

INGREDIENTS

- 16 Pounds asparagus spears
- 10 Tbsps. salt
- Boiling water

DIRECTIONS

1. In a large pot, cover the asparagus with the boiling water and add the salt. Boil for 3 minutes. Fill the sterilized jars loosely with the asparagus and liquid, leaving a 1 inch headspace.
2. Adjust the jar lids and process the jars for 30 minutes in a pressure canner at 10 pounds of pressure for a pressure canner with a weighted gauge, or 11 pounds if the pressure canner has a dial gauge.

Nutritions: Calories: 20 Cal; Protein: 2.2 g; Fat: 0.2 g; Carbs: 17 g

2. Lima Beans, Shelled

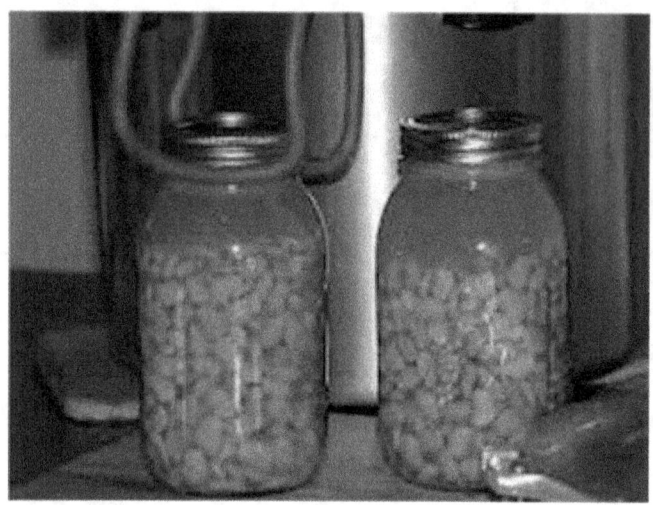

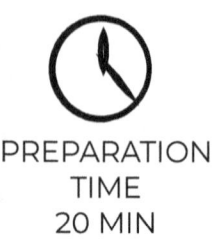

PREPARATION TIME
20 MIN

COOK TIME
50 MIN

SERVING
9 PINTS

INGREDIENTS

- *18 pounds lima beans, shelled*
- *10 tablespoons salt*
- *Boiling water*

DIRECTIONS

1. In a large pot, cover the beans with the boiling water and add the salt. Boil the beans for 10 minutes. Fill the sterilized jars loosely with beans and liquid, leaving a 1 inch headspace.
2. Adjust the jar lids and process the jars for 40 minutes in a pressure canner at 10 pounds of pressure for a pressure canner with a weighted gauge, or 11 pounds if the pressure canner has a dial gauge.

Nutritions: Calories: 88 Cal; Protein: 5.3 g; Fat: 0.7 g; Carbs: 15.7 g

3. White Potatoes: Cubed or Whole

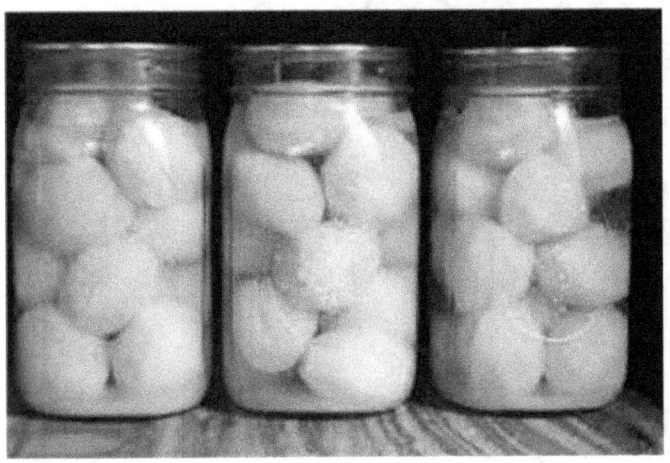

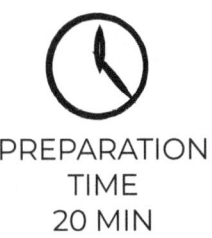

PREPARATION TIME
20 MIN

COOK TIME
45 MIN

SERVING
9 PINTS

INGREDIENTS

- Tbsp. salt
- Boiling water
- 13 Pounds potatoes

DIRECTIONS

1. Wash and peel the potatoes and place them in ascorbic acid solution, made up of 1 gallon of water and 1 cup of lemon juice, to prevent them from darkening. Drain the potatoes and allow to cook for 10 minutes in boiling salt water. You may use paper towels to drain them.
2. Fill the sterilized jars with the potatoes. Cover the potatoes with fresh boiling water, leaving a 1 inch headspace.
3. Process in a pressure canner for 35 minutes at 10 pounds of pressure for a pressure canner with a weighted gauge, or 11 pounds if the pressure canner has a dial gauge.

Nutritions: Calories: 117 Cal; Protein: 1.26 g; Fat: 0.08 g; Carbs: 17 g

4. Italian Style Stewed Tomatoes

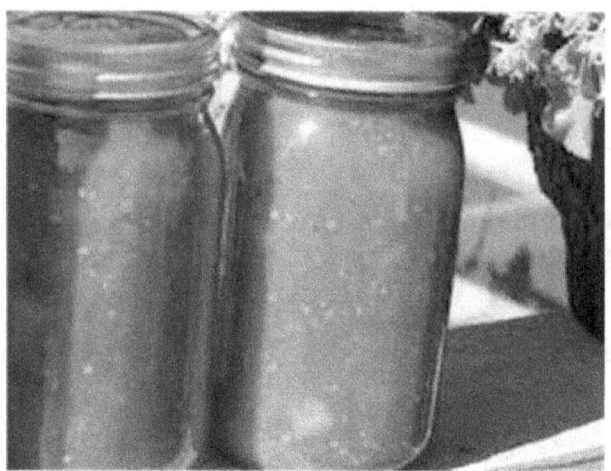

INGREDIENTS

- Quarts chopped tomatoes
- 1 Cup chopped onions
- 1/2 Cup chopped green peppers
- 4 Garlic cloves, minced
- 3 Tsps. Dry basil
- 1 Tsp. Dry oregano
- 4 Tsps. Sugar
- 1 Tsp. Salt
- 1 Tsp. Black pepper

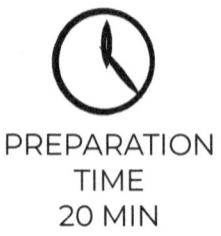

PREPARATION TIME
20 MIN

COOK TIME
25 MIN

SERVING
6 PINTS

DIRECTIONS

1. Place all of the ingredients in a large saucepan and bring to a boil. Let this mixture simmer for about 10 minutes, stirring occasionally.
2. Pack the sterilized jars with the hot tomato mixture, leaving a 1/2 inch head space. Remove any air bubbles, clean the rims and adjust lids.
3. Process the jars for 15 minutes in a pressure canner at 10 pounds of pressure for a pressure canner with a weighted gauge, or 11 pounds if the pressure canner has a dial gauge.

Nutritions: Calories: 40 Cal; Protein: 2 g; Fat: 0 g; Carbs: 22 g

5. Tomatoes: Whole

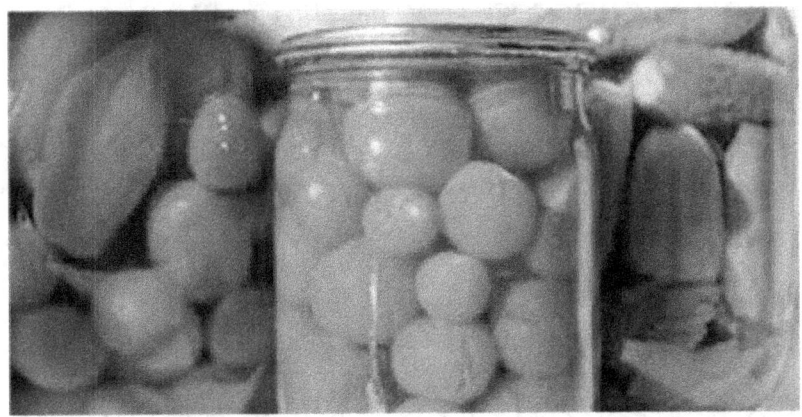

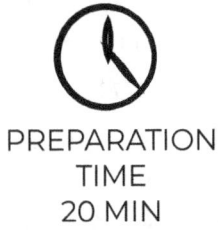

PREPARATION TIME
20 MIN

COOK TIME
45 MIN

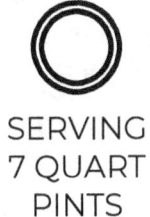

SERVING
7 QUART PINTS

INGREDIENTS

- *21 Pounds whole tomatoes, skinned*
- *4 Tbsps. salt*
- *3/4 Cup lemon juice, optional*
- *Boiling water*

DIRECTIONS

1. Place the tomatoes and the salt in a saucepan and cover with the water. Bring to a boil and cook for 5 minutes.
2. Pack sterilized jars with the tomatoes and the hot liquid, leaving a 1/2 inch head space. Remove any air bubbles, clean the rim and adjust lids.
3. If omitting the lemon juice, process the jars for 45 minutes in a pressure canner at 10 pounds of pressure for a pressure canner with a weighted gauge, or 11 pounds if the pressure canner has a dial gauge.
4. If using lemon juice, process the jars for 10 minutes in a boiling water bath.

Nutritions: Calories: 33 Cal; Protein: 1.3 g; Fat: 0.4 g; Carbs: 7.1 g

Tomato Canning 101

While some vegetables lose vital nutrients when exposed to high heat, tomatoes actually experience an increase in lycopene, a nutrient that devours 10 times more oxygenated free radicals in our bodies than vitamin E. Of course, heating does deplete some of the vitamin C found in tomatoes, but because we are using a pressure canner, we can process tomatoes for a shorter length of time to lessen the vitamin loss. So grab your clean jars and let's get to pressure canning these health-packed fruits in a variety of tasty ways.

Which Tomatoes Should I Choose?

There is no wrong tomato; they are all delicious in a jar! What it comes down to, however, is prep time and what you prefer to grow if you have a garden.

For my canning projects, I gravitate to Roma tomatoes, also called plum or oblong tomatoes, because of their thin skin and a more solid center. Using a Roma saves me from having to blanch the tomato and peel the skin and keeps my recipes from having an overabundance of liquid. I also use canning tomatoes, also known as globe, round, or beefsteak tomatoes. One year in particular, I had no choice but to use canning tomatoes because there just wasn't a good harvest for Romas due to the weather. At the end of the day, choose whatever tomato you enjoy eating, growing, or using in everyday cooking.

Preparing Tomatoes for Canning

When selecting tomatoes to preserve, make sure they are firm and not overly ripe. Do not preserve bruised, overly soft tomatoes or those that show signs of mold or yeast growth. Once you've gathered your bounty, here are some basic tips for tomato canning:

Adding Acid

Tomatoes are higher in acid when green; as enzymes ripen tomatoes into their luscious red color, their overall acidic value decreases. With the plethora of hybrids on the market and the natural pH fluctuation as a tomato ripens, it is always safest, when canning tomatoes, to increase their acid by adding bottled, not fresh, lemon juice (bottled lemon juice *has a much more standardized pH level). Below is a handy reference chart to help you determine how much lemon juice to add to your tomatoes before canning.*

TOMATO ACIDIFICATION	
JAR SIZE	**AMOUNT OF BOTTLED LEMON JUICE**
Half-pint (8 ounces)	1½ Teaspoons
Pint (16 ounces)	1 Tablespoon
Quart (32 ounces)	2 Tablespoons

6. Spiced Beets

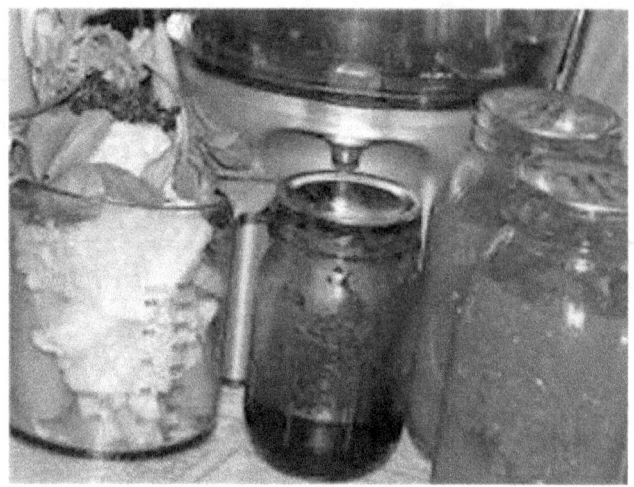

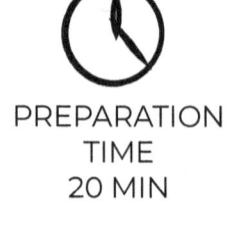

PREPARATION TIME 20 MIN

COOK TIME 25 MIN

SERVING 2 HALF PINTS

INGREDIENTS

- 1/4 Tsp. Salt
- 3/4 Tsp. Allspice
- 3/4 Tsp. Cloves
- 1/4 Stick cinnamon
- 1/4 Piece mace
- 1-1/2 Tsps. Celery seed
- 2 Cups cider vinegar, 5% acidity
- 1 Cup sugar
- 2 Pints beets

DIRECTIONS

1. Tie the salt and the spices in a thin cloth bag. Boil the vinegar, sugar, and spices for 15 minutes. Sterilize a quart jar for 15 minutes. Remove the jar from the water and pour in the vinegar mix. Fix the lid and set aside for 2 weeks.
2. Remove the spice bag. Cook fresh beets until tender but firm, and let cool. Peel the beets. Heat the vinegar and add 1/2 cup of the beet liquid. Add the beets and simmer for 15 minutes.
3. Pack into sterile jars, being sure the vinegar covers the beets. Remove air bubbles and adjust the lids. Process for 10 minutes in a boiling water bath.

Nutritions: Calories: Calories 174 Cal; Fat: 12 g; Carbs: 18 g; Protein 1 g

7. Spicy Carrots

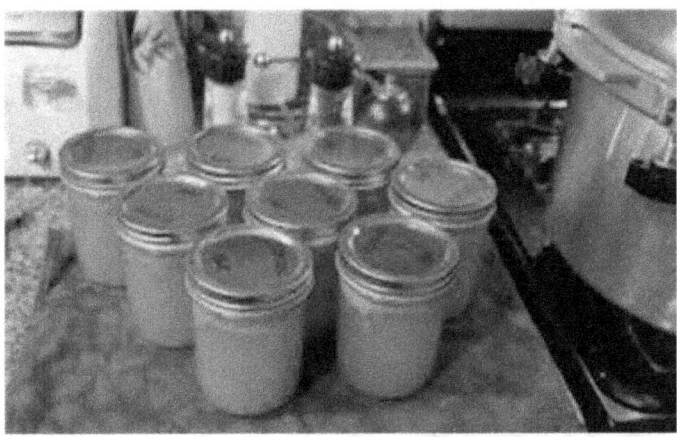

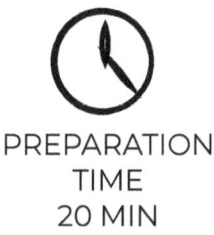

PREPARATION TIME
20 MIN

COOK TIME
30 MIN

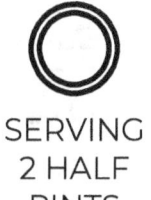

SERVING
2 HALF PINTS

INGREDIENTS

- 1/4 Tsp. Salt
- 3/4 Tsp. Allspice
- 3/4 Tsp. Cloves
- 1/4 Stick cinnamon
- 1/4 Piece mace
- 1-1/2 Tsps. Celery seed
- 2 Cups cider vinegar, 5% acidity
- 1 Cup sugar
- 2 Pints carrots

- 1/4 Tsp. Salt
- 3/4 Tsp. Allspice
- 3/4 Tsp. Cloves
- 1/4 Stick cinnamon
- 1/4 Piece mace
- 1-1/2 Tsps. Celery seed
- 2 Cups cider vinegar, 5% acidity
- 1 Cup sugar
- 2 Pints carrots

DIRECTIONS

1. Tie the salt and the spices in thin cloth bag. Boil the vinegar, sugar, and spices for 15 minutes. Sterilize a quart jar for about 15 minutes in boiling water. Remove the jar from the water and pour in the vinegar mix. Fix the lid and set aside for 2 weeks.
2. Remove the spice bag. Cook fresh carrots until tender but firm, and let cool. Heat the vinegar and add 1/2 cup of the carrot liquid. Add the carrots and simmer for 15 minutes.
3. Pack into sterile jars, being sure the vinegar covers the carrots. Remove air bubbles and adjust the lids. Process 10 minutes in a boiling water bath.

Nutritions: Calories: 71 Cal; Fat: 1 g; Carbs: 16 g; Protein 2 g

8. Sweet Corn Salad

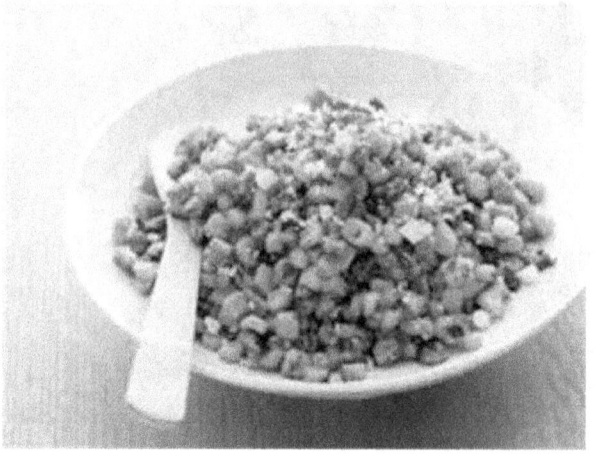

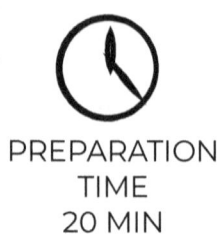

PREPARATION TIME
20 MIN

COOK TIME
55 MIN

SERVING
5 PINTS

INGREDIENTS

- Cups corn kernels
- 2 Green bell peppers
- 1 Red bell pepper
- 4 Onions (yellow or white)
- 1 Tsp. Celery seed
- 1 Tbsp. Dry mustard
- 2-2/3 Cups of white wine vinegar
- 2-2/3 Cups of sugar
- 1/2 Tsp. Ground turmeric

DIRECTIONS

1. Halve seeds, and peppers to de-rib.
2. Coarsely chop, to the size of a kernel of corn.
3. Chop them the same size as the onions.
4. Throw all the ingredients into a heavy kettle or pot.
5. Heat to a slow boil and continue cooking for ten minutes at this temperature, or until the vegetables are tender.
6. Pour into hot jars, ensuring all jars receive equal amounts of liquid.
7. Wipe the rims and screw them on the lids and rings.

Pressure Canner Process: Pints: 55 Minutes; Quarts 85 Minutes

Nutritions: Calories: 149 Cal; Protein: 3.1 g; Fat: 8.1 g; Carbs: 19 g

9. Garden Vegetable Medley

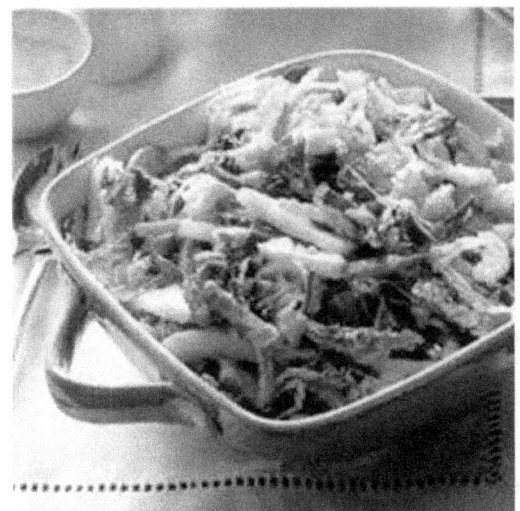

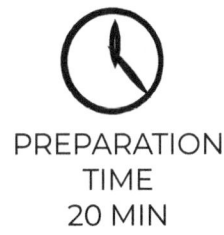
PREPARATION TIME
20 MIN

COOK TIME
30 MIN

SERVING
4 PINTS

INGREDIENTS

- 2 Cups carrots
- 2 Cups green beans
- 2 Cups celery
- 2 Cups cauliflower
- 2 Cups chopped fennel
- 2 Cups boiling onions
- 2 Cups green bell peppers
- 4 Cups white vinegar
- 1/3 Cup olive oil
- 1/2 Cup salt (kosher)
- 1/2 Cup sugar

DIRECTIONS

1. Prepare all the vegetables into pieces of similar size.
2. Set aside in single containers.
3. In a non-reactive pot or bath, add the vinegar, butter, salt, and sugar.
4. Take to boil.
5. In this order, add vegetables, allowing liquid to return to a boil between each: carrots, beans, celery, cauliflower, fennel, and finally, the peeled, whole ointments.
6. Cook only until tender-crisp carrots are in.
7. Attach the peppers and cook another minute or less, just to heat through the peppers.
8. Pour into hot jars, ensuring all jars receive equal amounts of liquid.
9. Wipe the rims and screw them on lids and rings.

Pressure Canner Process: pints: 25 Minutes; Quarts: 30 Minutes

Nutritions: Calories: 70 Cal; Protein: 2 g; Fat: 0.5 g; Carbs: 14 g

10. Mixed Vegetables, Italian Style

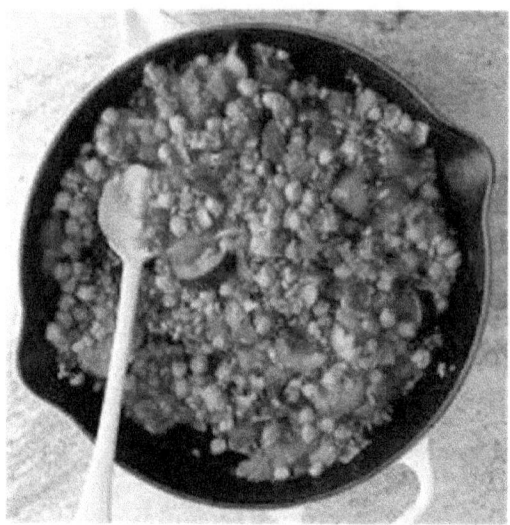

INGREDIENTS

PREPARATION TIME 20 MIN

COOK TIME 30 MIN

SERVING 4 PINTS

- 4 Cups tomatoes, chopped
- 1 Cup carrots, chopped
- 1 Cup celery, chopped
- 1 Cup green beans, cut into 1-inch pieces
- 1 Large bell pepper
- 3 Cups Zucchini, chopped
- 1 Cup boiling onions
- 1/2 Cup olive oil
- 1-1/2 Cup salt (kosher)
- 1 Cup sugar
- 2 Cups white vinegar
- 8 Fresh mint leaves
- 1 Cup fresh basil leaves

DIRECTIONS

1. Cook the tomatoes at low heat until they turn into a thick purée.
2. To remove skin and seeds, press through the food mill and put it in a clean pan.
3. Add olive oil, salt, sugar, and 1 1/4 cup vinegar.
4. Take to boil.
5. Add carrots, celery, beans, and (peeled) onions and cook for another five minutes.
6. Add the peppers, zucchini, sage, basil, and nutmeg; cook for 3-5 minutes until vegetables are tender-crisp.
7. Take the pan off the fire.
8. Heat the remaining vinegar to a boil in another bowl, and cook the slices of cucumber in it until tender, about ten minutes.
9. Drain the cucumbers and add them to the first saucepan.
10. If used, add capers.
11. Pour into hot jars, ensuring all jars receive equal amounts of liquid.
12. Wipe the rims and screw them on lids and rings.

Pressure Canner Process: Pints: 25 Minutes; Quarts: 30 Minutes

Nutritions: 7.5 Cal; Protein: 0.1 g; Fat: 0.6 g; Carbs: 0.5 g

Chapter 11.
Meat and Poultry Recipes

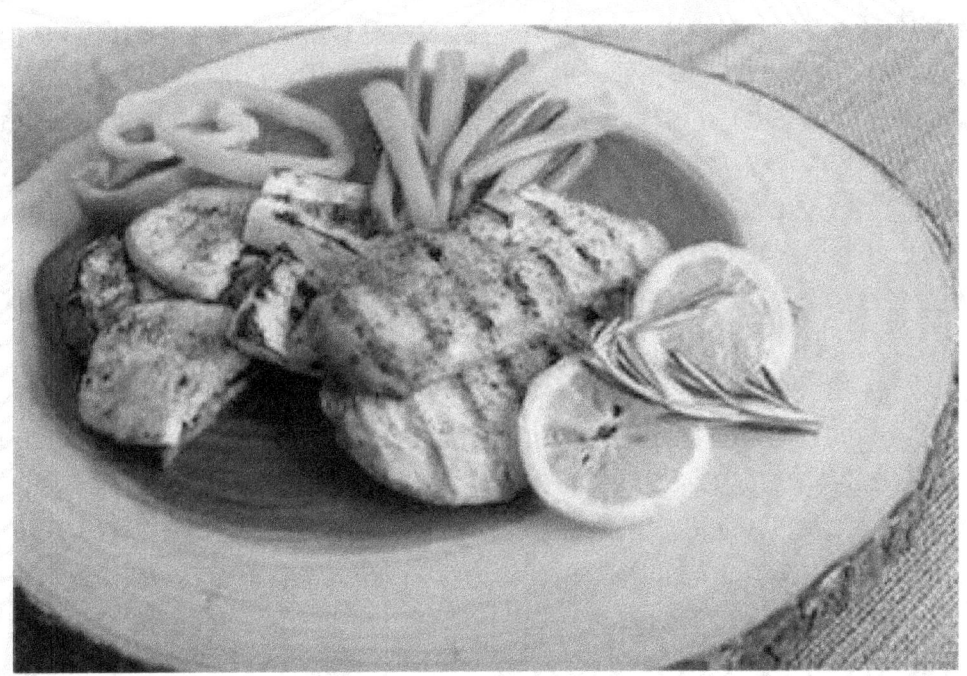

Poultry
Home-canned chicken is the perfect starter for so many quick, healthy recipes you'll wonder why you didn't think of this sooner. Simply heat and add seasonings to create meals like chicken curry soup, tacos, enchiladas and chicken Alfredo. Home-canned chicken is even great to take for camping. The protein-packed possibilities are endless!

PREPARING POULTRY FOR CANNING

While the chart below gives you the math behind what fits into a jar, make sure to use the following tips when filling a jar:
1. Remove the excess fat and skin from breasts and thighs.

2. Keep the bones in legs and thighs if preferred.
3. Add cool water when raw packing or hot broth when hot packing for the best results.
4. Pre-cook ground poultry and drain any excess liquid or fat.
5. Ground poultry can be canned loose, in patties, or in links.
6. Always give each jar 1¼ inches of headspace when filling.
7. Always wipe the jar rim and rings with a warm wet washcloth, dipped in distilled white vinegar.
8. If you raise chickens, be sure to chill dressed poultry for 6 to 12 hours before canning.
9. Adding water to raw-packed chicken is a preference. Meat without the addition of water will make its own broth in the jar while it cooks during processing; however, it is not enough broth to fully cover all the meat. The old instruction that told us not to add water when raw packing was for the fear that the meat would overproduce a liquid, which would then cause grease to get onto the jar rim and prevent a lid seal from forming. As long as you maintain a 1¼ inch headspace and wipe each jar rim with distilled white vinegar, you have sufficiently eliminated the possibility of the lid not sealing. While it is still acceptable to skip the added water when raw packing, I personally prefer to add water so I have the choice to use the broth in the jar during the meal creation. Plus, when I add water during raw packing, I can be sure the meat is fully covered with enough liquid to prevent oxidization, which discolors and dries out the uncovered meat.

POULTRY PROCESSING CHART					
TYPE	PREPA-RATION	QUANTITY	PACK TYPE	AMOUNT PER PINT	AMOUNT PER QUART
Boneless Skinless Breasts	Cut Into 2 inch Pieces	22 To 28	Raw	2 Breasts	4 Breasts
Boneless Skinless Thighs	Cut Into 2 inch Pieces	40 To 55	Raw	4 Thighs	8 Thighs

Canning and Preserving for Beginners

Breast, Bone-In	Whole, Skin Removed	14	Raw	1 Breast	2 Breasts
Thighs, Bone-In	Whole, Skin Removed	35 To 42	Raw	3 Or 4 Thighs	5 Or 6 Thighs
Legs, Bone-In	Whole, Skin Removed	42	Raw	3 Legs	6 Legs
Ground	Cooked, Fat Drained	14 Pounds	Hot	1 Pound	2 Pounds

TYPE	Yield In Pints	Yield In Quarts	Processing Time For Quarts	Processing Time For Pints	Psi Dial Gauge*	Psi Weighted Gauge*
Boneless Skinless Breasts	7	14	1 Hr. 30 Min	1 Hr. 15 Min	11 Psi	10 Psi
Boneless Skinless Thighs	7	14	1 Hr. 30 Min	1 Hr. 15 Min	11 Psi	10 Psi
Breast, Bone-In	7	14	1 Hr. 15 Min	1 Hr. 5 Min	11 Psi	10 Psi
Thighs, Bone-In	7	14	1 Hr. 15 Min	1 Hr. 5 Min	11 Psi	10 Psi
Legs, Bone-In	7	14	1 Hr. 15 Min	1 Hr. 5 Min	11 Psi	10 Psi
Ground	7	14	1 Hr. 30 Min	1 Hr. 15 Min	11 Psi	10 Psi

*For elevations above 1,000 feet, check a Pressure Canning Altitude Chart to safely increase the PSI.

PORK

Home-canned pork is another perfect meat to have at the ready. I will typically can pork butt when it's on sale, so I have fully cooked pork shoulder, or butt, available when I am crunched for time and need to get a pulled pork meal on the table. I will also pressure-can ground pork when there is a huge sale, which saves me on freezer space and gives me a healthy alternative to ground beef.

PREPARING PORK FOR CANNING

Use this chart to determine how much pork you need for canning, and use the following tips when filling the jars:

1. Remove excess fat, silver skin and gristle, but keep marbleized fat to prevent drying out.
2. Brown all sides in fat and seasonings prior to filling jars for best results.
3. Precook ground pork and drain any excess liquid or fat.
4. Ground pork can be canned loose, in patties, or in links.
5. Always give each jar 1¼ inches of headspace when filling.
6. Always wipe the jar rim and screw a thread with a warm washcloth dipped in distilled white vinegar.

PORK PROCESSING CHART					
CUT	PREPARATION	QUANTITY	PACK TYPE	AMOUNT PER PINT	AMOUNT PER QUART
Tenderloin	Cut Into 2 inch Pieces	14 Pounds	Raw	1 Pound	2 Pounds
Pork Shoulder	Cut Into 2 inch Pieces, Browned	14 Pounds	Hot	1 Pound	2 Pounds
Pork Butt	Cut Into 2 inch Pieces, Browned	14 Pounds	Hot	1 Pound	2 Pounds

| Boneless Pork Chops | Cut Into 2 inch Pieces, Browned | 14 Pounds | Hot | 1 Pound | 2 Pounds |
| Ground | Cooked, Fat Drained | 14 Pounds | Hot | 1 Pound | 2 Pounds |

Cut	Yield in Pints	Yield in Quarts	Processing Time For Quarts	Processing Time For Pints	Psi Dial Gauge*	Psi Weighted Gauge*
Tenderloin	7	14	1 Hr. 30 Min	1 Hr. 15 Min	11 PSI	10 PSI
Pork Shoulder	7	14	1 Hr. 30 Min	1 Hr. 15 Min	11 Psi	10 Psi
Pork Butt	7	14	1 Hr. 30 Min	1 Hr. 15 Min	11 Psi	10 Psi
Boneless Pork Chops	7	14	1 Hr. 30 Min	1 Hr. 15 Min	11 Psi	10 Psi
Ground	7	14	1 Hr. 30 Min	1 Hr. 15 Min	11 Psi	10 Psi

* For elevations above 1,000 feet, check a Pressure Canning Altitude Chart to safely increase the PSI.

BEEF

Having jars of precooked roast beef, stew meat, beef tips, and ground beef saves me loads of time when planning and creating meals. Before canning, I like to preseason beef with salt, pepper, garlic, and onions or one of my favorite spice blends to give the meat a leg up on flavor. For instance, if you season your ground beef with the Taco Seasoning Spice Blend before canning, you've got a taco night, or an easy-to-pack lunch, ready to go at a moment's notice.

PREPARING BEEF FOR CANNING

While the chart below gives you the math behind what fits into a jar, make sure to use the following tips when filling a jar:

1. Remove excess fat, silver skin and gristle, but keep marbleized fat to prevent drying out.
2. Brown all sides in fat and seasonings prior to filling jars for best results.
3. Precook ground beef and drain any excess liquid or fat.
4. Ground beef can be canned loose or in patties.
5. Always give each jar 1¼ inches of headspace when filling.
6. Always wipe the jar rims and screw a thread with a warm washcloth dipped in distilled white vinegar.
7. Beef sold for stew is typically chuck, or round roasts cut into 1½ inch pieces. Bottom and eye cuts, also known as round, are typically leaner than a chuck roast, which includes cuts from the shoulder, leg, and butt. When cutting into bite-sized pieces, cut to a size you would feel comfortable seeing on the end of your fork or spoon.

BEEF PROCESSING CHART					
CUT	PREPARATION	QUANTITY	PACK TYPE	AMOUNT PER PINT	AMOUNT PER QUART
Chuck Steak	Cut Into 2 inch Pieces, Browned	14 Pounds	Hot	1 Pound	2 Pounds
Round Roast	Cut Into 2 inch Pieces, Browned	14 Pounds	Hot	1 Pound	2 Pounds
Stew Meat/ Beef Tips	Cut Into 2 inch Pieces, Browned	14 Pounds	Hot	1 Pound	2 Pounds

Canning and Preserving for Beginners

Cut	Yield in Pints	Yield in Quarts	Processing Time For Quarts	Processing Time For Pints	Psi Dial Gauge*	Psi Weighted Gauge*
Chuck Steak	7	14	1 Hr. 30 Min	1 Hr. 15 Min	11 Psi	10 Psi
Round Roast	7	14	1 Hr. 30 Min	1 Hr. 15 Min	11 Psi	10 Psi
Stew Meat/ Beef Tips	7	14	1 Hr. 30 Min	1 Hr. 15 Min	11 Psi	10 Psi
Ground	7	14	1 Hr. 30 Min	1 Hr. 15 Min	11 Psi	10 Psi

For elevations above 1,000 feet, check a Pressure Canning Altitude Chart to safely increase the PSI.

11. Dehydrated Candied Bacon

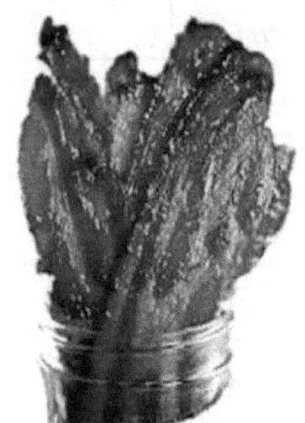

INGREDIENTS

- 1 lb. Bacon, thinly sliced
- 2 Cups sugar
- ¾ Water
- 1Tbsp. Lemon juice

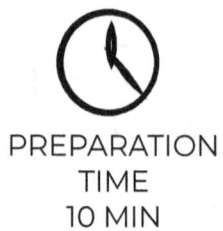

PREPARATION TIME
10 MIN

COOK TIME
8 H DEHYDRATION

SERVING
10

DIRECTIONS

1. Combine your sugar and water into a stock pan and place to boil for about 5minutes.
2. Add in your bacon, and set the strips on the dehydrator tray, place in the dehydrator and leave to fully dry at 135 degrees for about 10 – 12 hours.
3. Enjoy!

Nutritions: Calories: 102 Cal; Protein: 0 g; Fat: 0 g; Carbs: 27 g

12. Soy Marinated Salmon Jerky

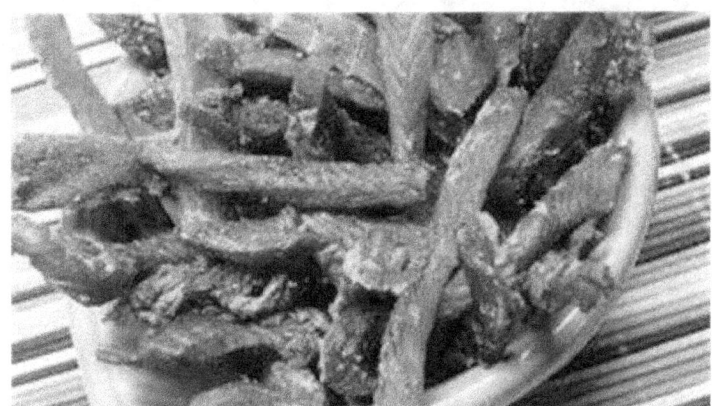

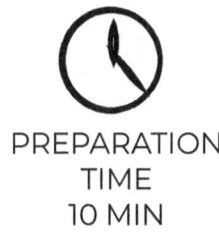

PREPARATION TIME
10 MIN

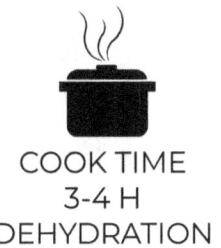

COOK TIME
3-4 H
DEHYDRATION

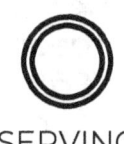

SERVING
2

INGREDIENTS

- 1 lbs. Boneless salmon fillet
- Salt and pepper to taste
- ½ Cup apple cider vinegar
- 2 Tablespoons low-sodium soy sauce
- 1 Tablespoon fresh lemon juice
- 2 Teaspoons paprika
- ½ Teaspoon garlic powder

DIRECTIONS

1. Freeze the salmon for about 30 minutes until it is firm.
2. Meanwhile, whisk together the apple cider vinegar, soy sauce, and lemon juice in a mixing bowl.
3. Add the paprika and garlic powder then stir well.
4. Season the salmon with salt and pepper to taste, then remove the skin.
5. Slice the salmon into ¼ inch thick strips, then place them in a bowl or glass dish.
6. Pour in the marinade, turning to coat, and then cover with plastic and chill for 12 hours.
7. Drain the salmon slices and place them on paper towels to soak up the extra liquid.
8. Spread the salmon slices on your dehydrator trays in a single layer.
9. Dry for 3 to 4 hours at 145°F (63°C) until it is dried, but still tender and chewy.
10. Cool the salmon jerky completely, then store in airtight containers in a cool, dark location.

Nutritions: Calories: 203 Cal; Protein: 0 g; Fat: 0 g; Carbs: 27 g

13. Teriyaki Beef Jerky

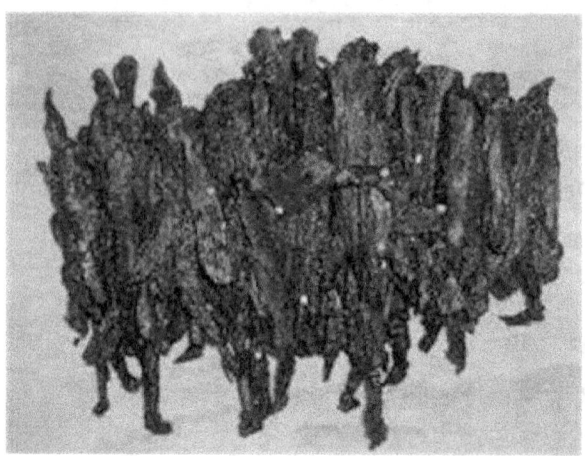

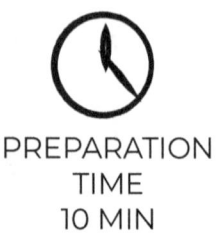

PREPARATION TIME
10 MIN

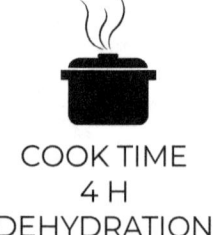

COOK TIME
4 H
DEHYDRATION

SERVING
2

INGREDIENTS

- 2 ½ to 3 lbs. Boneless beef sirloin
- Salt and pepper to taste
- ¼ Cup low-sodium soy sauce
- ¼ Cup light brown sugar, packed
- 2 Tablespoons liquid smoke
- 1 Teaspoon cider vinegar

DIRECTIONS

1. Whisk together the soy sauce, sugar, liquid smoke and cider vinegar in a mixing bowl.
2. Trim the fat from the beef and cut it into ¼ inch thick strips.
3. Season the beef with salt and pepper to taste, then add to the bowl with the marinade.
4. Toss to coat, then cover with plastic and chill for 24 hours.
5. Spread the meat slices on your dehydrator trays in a single layer.
6. Dry for 4 hours at 145 °F (63 °C) until it is dried, but still tender and chewy.
7. Cool the jerky completely, and then store it in airtight containers in a cool, dark location.

Nutritions: Carbs: 32 g; Fat: 11 g; Protein: 24 g; Sodium: 3 mg; Calories: 298 Cal

14. Pot Roast in a Jar

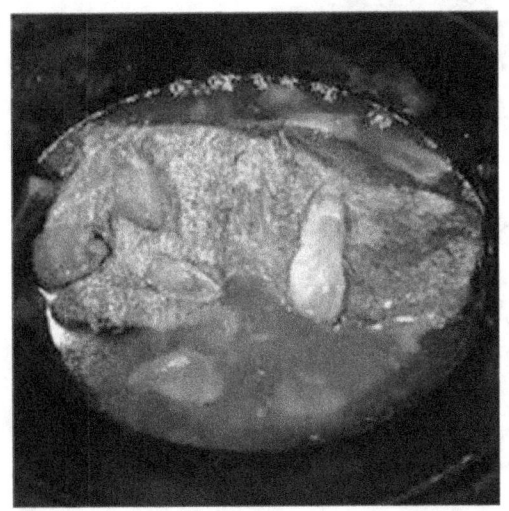

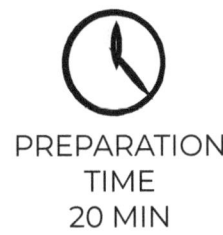
PREPARATION TIME
20 MIN

COOK TIME
50 MIN

SERVING
6

INGREDIENTS

- 2 Pounds stewing beef, cut into chunks
- 1 Cup chopped onions
- 2 Teaspoons dried thyme
- 2 Cloves of garlic, minced
- 2 Bay leaves
- 1 Cup beef broth
- 1 Cup dry red wine
- 2 Teaspoons salt
- 1 Teaspoon ground black pepper
- 1 Cup chopped carrots
- 1 Cup diced potatoes
- ½ Cup chopped celery

DIRECTIONS

1. Sterilize the jars in a pressure canner as indicated in the general guidelines of this book. Allow the jars to cool.
2. Place the beef in a pot and add in the onions, thyme, garlic, bay leaves, broth, and wine. Season with salt and black pepper. Close the lid and turn on the heat. Bring to a boil for 10 minutes and allow to simmer for 10 minutes.
3. Add in the vegetables and simmer for another 5 minutes. Turn off the heat.
4. Transfer the mixture to sterilized jars.
5. Remove the air bubbles and close the lid.
6. Place the jars in the pressure canner. Place it in a pressure canner and process for 25 minutes.

Nutritions: Calories: 234 Cal; Protein: 34.2 g; Sugar: 2 g; Fat: 6.2 g; Carbs: 9.3 g

15. Canned Beef Stroganoff

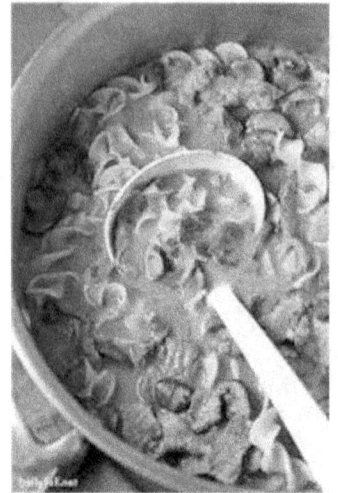

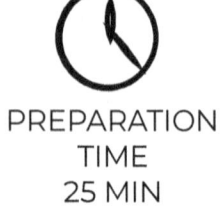

PREPARATION TIME
25 MIN

COOK TIME
50 MIN

SERVING
6

INGREDIENTS

- 1 Teaspoon black pepper
- 2 Teaspoons salt
- 2 Teaspoons thyme
- 2 Teaspoons parsley
- 4 Tablespoons Worcestershire sauce
- 2 Cloves of garlic, minced
- 1 Cup mushrooms, sliced
- 1 Cup onion, chopped
- 2 Pounds stewing beef, cut into chunks
- 4 Cups beef broth

DIRECTIONS

1. Sterilize the jars in a pressure canner as indicated in the general guidelines of this book. Allow the jars to cool.
2. Add all ingredients in a pot and bring it to a boil for 5 minutes. Reduce the heat and allow it to simmer for another 20 minutes. Turn off the heat and allow to cool slightly.
3. Transfer the mixture to sterilized jars.
4. Remove the air bubbles and close the lid.
5. Place the jars in the pressure canner. Place it in a pressure canner and process for 25 minutes.

Nutritions: Calories: 207 Cal; Protein: 33.5 g; Fat: 6.1 g; Carbs: 5.1 g; Sugar: 1.2g

16. Canned Ground Beef

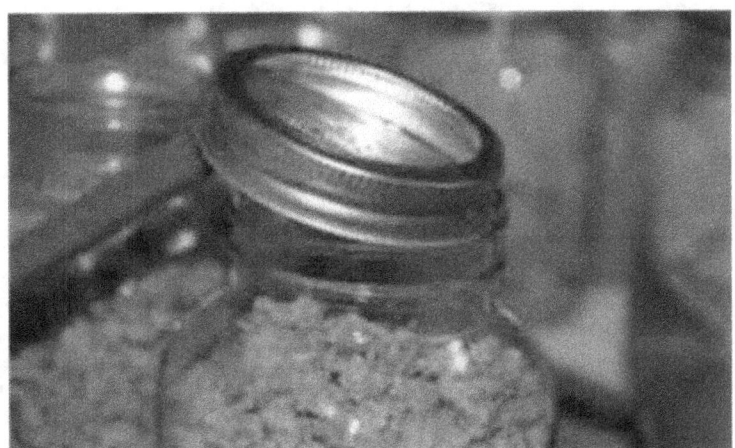

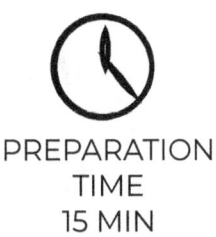

PREPARATION TIME
15 MIN

COOK TIME
35 MIN

SERVING
5

INGREDIENTS

- 2 Pounds ground beef
- 3 Cups water
- Pickling salt

DIRECTIONS

1. Sterilize the jars in a pressure canner as indicated in the general guidelines of this book. Allow the jars to cool.
2. Place beef in a skillet and sauté the meat for 10 minutes until browned.
3. Pack the meat loosely in the sterilized jars. Set aside.
4. In a pan, bring water to a boil and add ½ teaspoon canning salt per pint of water. Stir to dissolve the salt.
5. Pour the canning liquid over the beef and leave a 1 inch headspace.
6. Remove the air bubbles and close the lid.
7. Place the jars in the pressure canner. Place in a pressure canner and process for 25 minutes.

Nutritions: Calories: 392 Cal; Protein: 48.3 g; Sugar: 0 g; Fat: 20.2 g; Carbs: 0.6 g

17. Canned Chipotle Beef

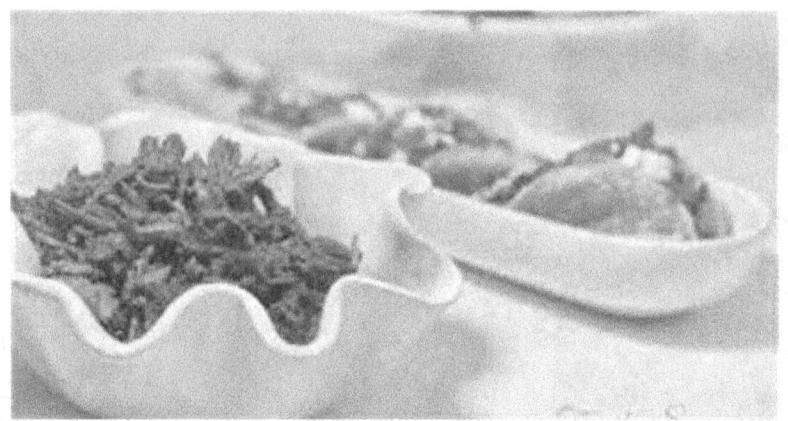

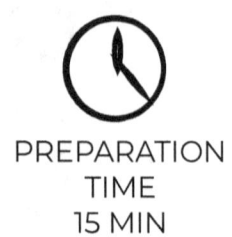

PREPARATION TIME 15 MIN

COOK TIME 48 MIN

SERVING 6

INGREDIENTS

- 2 Pounds beef brisket, cut into chunks
- 2 Teaspoons salt
- 8 Cloves of garlic, minced
- 2 Cups onion, chopped
- 2 Teaspoons oregano
- ½ Cup coriander
- 2 Chipotle chilies, chipped
- 4 Cups beef broth

DIRECTIONS

1. Sterilize the jars in a pressure canner as indicated in the general guidelines of this book. Allow the jars to cool.
2. Place the beef in a pot and season with salt. Turn on the heat and sear all sides for 3 minutes. Stir in the garlic and onion. Cook for another minute. Add in the rest of the ingredients.
3. Close the lid and allow the meat to simmer for 20 minutes on medium heat. Turn off the heat and allow the mixture to slightly cool.
4. Transfer the mixture to the jars.
5. Remove the air bubbles and close the lid.
6. Place the jars in the pressure canner. Place in a pressure canner and process for 25 minutes.

Nutritions: Calories: 322 Cal; Protein: 22.9 g; Sugar: 1.7 g; Fat: 22 g; Carbs: 5.4 g

18. Canned Goulash

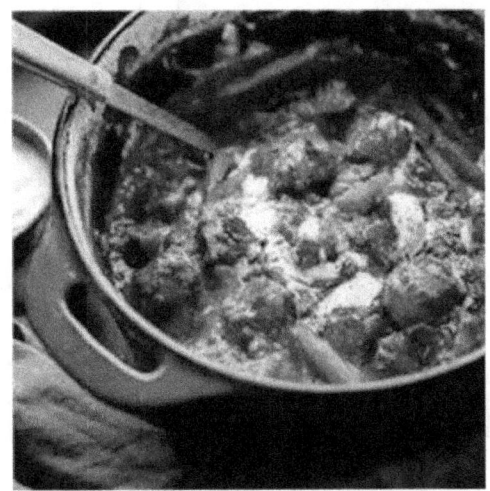

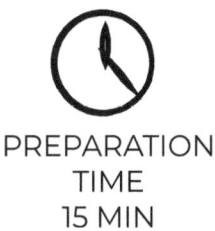

PREPARATION TIME
15 MIN

COOK TIME
45 MIN

SERVING
5

INGREDIENTS

- 4 Pounds stewing beef, cut into chunks
- Peppercorns
- 3 Bay leaves
- 2 Teaspoons caraway seeds
- 1/3 Cup vegetable oil
- 3 Onions, chopped
- 1 Tablespoon salt
- 6 Celery stalks, chopped
- 4 Carrots, peeled and chopped
- 2 Teaspoons mustard powder
- 1 ½ Cups water
- 1/3 Cup vinegar

DIRECTIONS

1. Sterilize the jars in a pressure canner as indicated in the general guidelines of this book. Allow the jars to cool.
2. Place the meat in a bowl and add in the peppercorns, bay leaves, and caraway seeds. Massage the beef and allow to marinate for an hour in the fridge.
3. Heat oil in a saucepan over medium flame. Sauté the onions for one minute until fragrant and stir in the seasoned beef. Season with salt to taste before adding the rest of the ingredients.
4. Close the lid and bring to a boil for 5 minutes. Simmer for 15 minutes. Turn off the heat and allow to cool slightly.
5. Transfer the mixture to the jars.
6. Remove the air bubbles and close the lid.
7. Place the jars in the pressure canner. Place in a pressure canner and process for 25 minutes.

Nutritions: Calories: 627 Cal; Protein: 80.9 g; Sugar: 4.4 g; Fat: 29.2 g; Carbs: 11.2 g

CANNING AND PRESERVING FOR BEGINNERS

19. Canned Chicken and Gravy

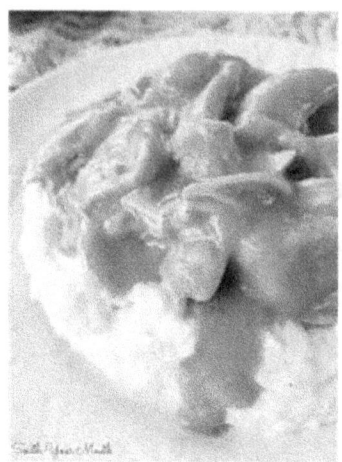

INGREDIENTS

- 1 Cup chopped onion
- 1 Cup chopped celery
- 1 Cup diced potatoes
- 2 Pounds boneless chicken breasts
- 2 Teaspoons salt
- 2 Teaspoons poultry seasoning
- 4 Tablespoons white wine
- Enough chicken stock to fill the jars

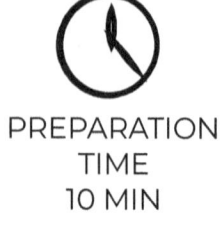

PREPARATION TIME
10 MIN

COOK TIME
35 MIN

SERVING
5

DIRECTIONS

1. Sterilize the jars in a pressure canner as indicated in the general guidelines of this book. Allow the jars to cool.
2. Place all ingredients in a saucepan and allow to simmer for 10 minutes over medium high heat.
3. Put the chicken and vegetables into the jars. Pour over enough broth to cover the chicken. Leave a ½ inch headspace.
4. Remove the air bubbles and close the lid.
5. Place the jars in the pressure canner. Place in a pressure canner and process for 25 minutes.

Nutritions: Calories: 562 Cal; Protein: 77.7 g; Sugar: 0 g; Fat: 22.2 g; Carbs: 7.1 g

20. Canned Meatballs

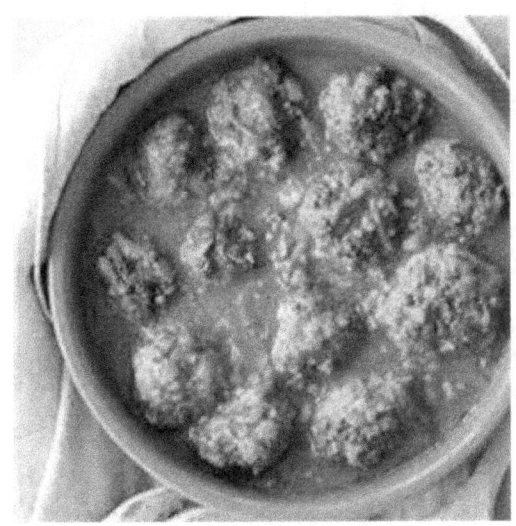

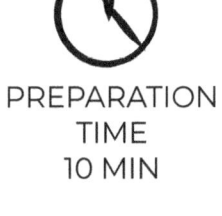

PREPARATION TIME
10 MIN

COOK TIME
30 MIN

SERVING
5

INGREDIENTS

- 2 Pounds ground meat
- Herbs of your choice
- 2 Teaspoons salt
- Enough tomato juice to cover the meatballs

DIRECTIONS

1. Sterilize the jars in a pressure canner as indicated in the general guidelines of this book. Allow the jars to cool.
2. Place meat in a bowl and stir in the herbs and salt. Mix until well combined.
3. Boil enough water in a saucepan. Make balls out of the ground meat mixture and gently drop them into the boiling water. Allow to cook for 5 minutes, then strain the meatballs.
4. Gently pack the meatballs inside the sterilized jars. Pour in enough tomato juice over the meatballs. Leave an inch of headspace.
5. Remove the air bubbles and close the lid.
6. Place the jars in the pressure canner. Place it in a pressure canner and process for 25 minutes.

Nutritions: Calories: 272 Cal; Protein: 35.8 g; Sugar: 0 g; Fat: 14 g; Carbs: 0.8 g

21. Canned Pork

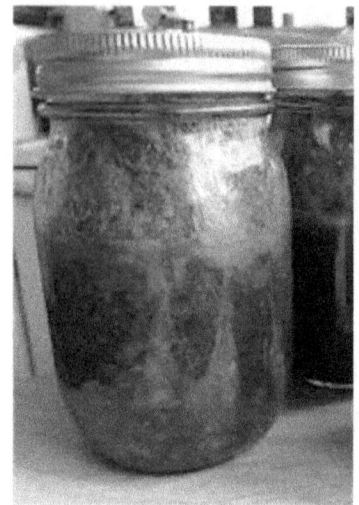

INGREDIENTS

- 2 Pounds pork chops, boneless
- Canning salt
- Water

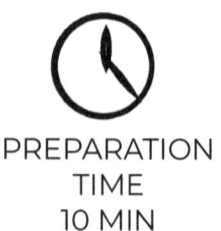

PREPARATION TIME
10 MIN

COOK TIME
40 MIN

SERVING
5 PINTS

DIRECTIONS

1. Sterilize the jars in a pressure canner as indicated in the general guidelines of this book. Allow the jars to cool.
2. Place the pork chops in boiling water and allow it to simmer for 15 minutes. Strain the cooked pork and pack them in the sterilized jars.
3. In a pan, bring water to a boil and add ½ teaspoon canning salt per pint of water. Stir to dissolve the salt.
4. Pour pickling solution into the jar to cover the pork. Leave an inch of headspace.
5. Remove the air bubbles and close the lid.
6. Place the jars in the pressure canner. Place it in a pressure canner and process for 25 minutes.

Nutritions: Calories: 379 Cal; Protein: 46.7 g; Carbs: 0 g; Fat: 20.1g; Sugar: 0g

22. Canned Turkey

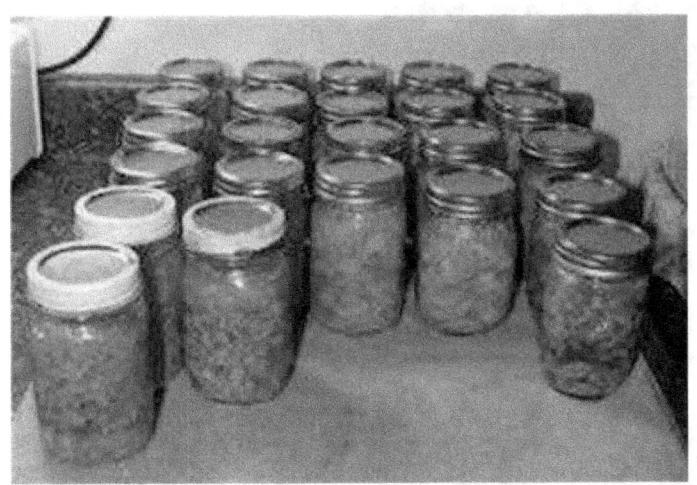

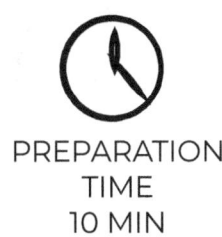

PREPARATION TIME
10 MIN

COOK TIME
35 MIN

SERVING
5

INGREDIENTS

- 2 Pounds turkey breasts, sliced into bite-sized pieces
- Canning salt
- Water

DIRECTIONS

1. Sterilize the jars in a pressure canner as indicated in the general guidelines of this book. Allow the jars to cool.
2. Place the turkey breasts in boiling water and allow to simmer for 10 minutes. Strain the cooked turkey and pack them in the sterilized jars.
3. In a pan, bring water to a boil and add ½ teaspoon canning salt per pint of water. Stir to dissolve the salt.
4. Pour pickling solution into the jar to cover the turkey. Leave an inch of headspace.
5. Remove the air bubbles and close the lid.
6. Place the jars in the pressure canner. Place in a pressure canner and process for 25 minutes.

Nutritions: Calories: 285 Cal; Protein: 39.7 g; Sugar: 0 g; Fat: 12.7 g; Carbs: 0 g

23. Canned Chili

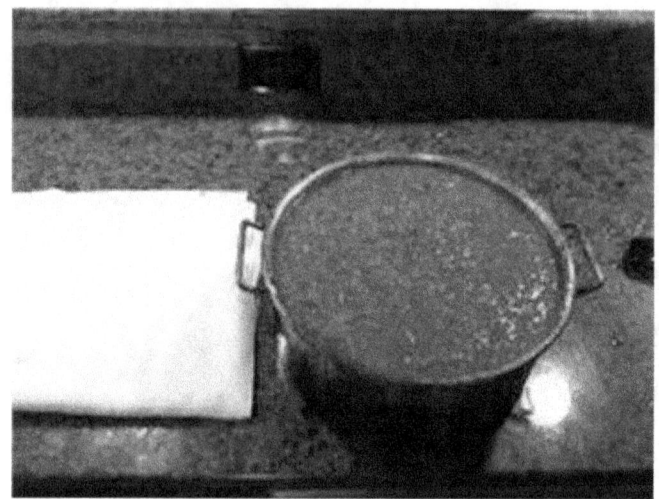

INGREDIENTS

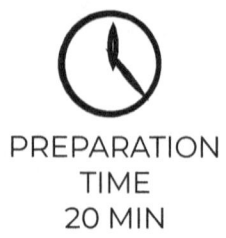

PREPARATION TIME
20 MIN

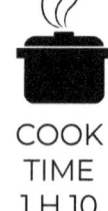

COOK TIME
1 H 10

SERVING
6

- 3 Cups dry kidney beans, soaked overnight and drained
- 2 Pounds ground beef
- 1 Cup onion, chopped
- 1 Cup pepper, seeded and chopped
- 4 Cups tomatoes, chopped
- 1 Tablespoon chili pepper, seeded and chopped

DIRECTIONS

1. Sterilize the jars in a pressure canner as indicated in the general guidelines of this book. Allow the jars to cool.
2. Place the beans in a pot and boil for 30 minutes. Drain the beans.
3. In a clean pot, put the cooked beans and the rest of the ingredients. Cook for another 20 minutes.
4. Transfer the mixture into the sterilized jars. Leave an inch of headspace.
5. Remove the air bubbles and close the lid.
6. Place the jars in the pressure canner. Place in a pressure canner and process for 25 minutes.

Nutritions: Calories: 412 Cal; Protein: 43.8 g; Carbs: 10.4g; Fat: 20.9g; Sugar: 4.1g

Chapter 12.
Stock, Broths Soup and Stew Recipes

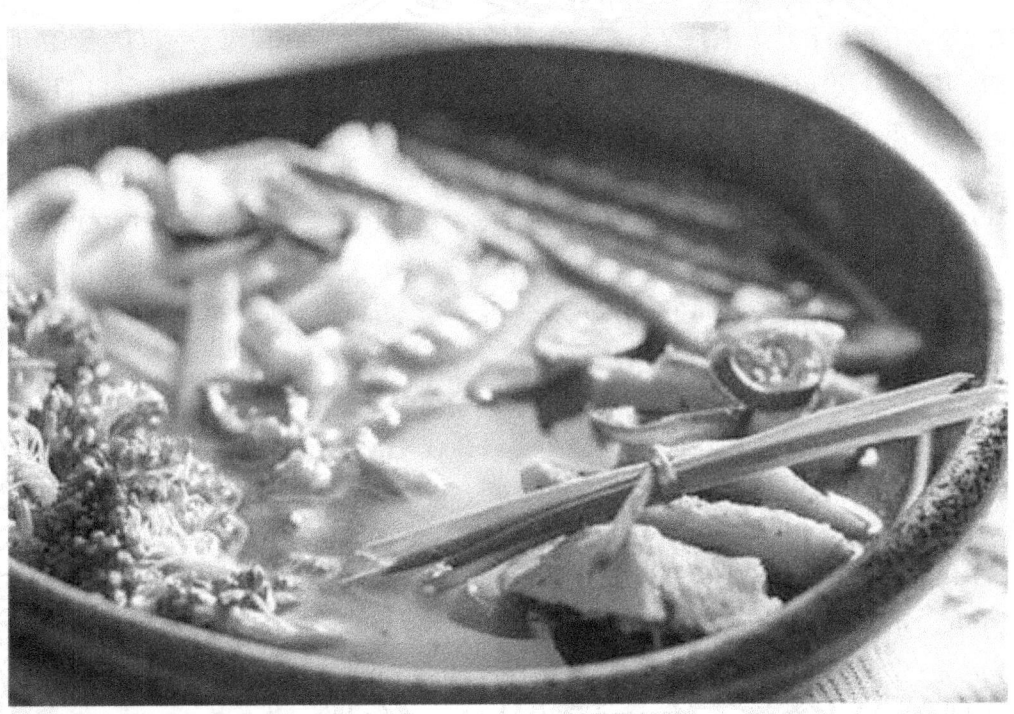

MAKING CANNING BROTH

Meat and poultry should be canned in a broth made from the bones of the type of animal being canned.

For poultry, remove as much of the meat from the carcass as you can, place the bones in a pot of water and cook on medium heat for 45 minutes. Take the bones out and remove any remaining meat from the bones. Add the meat back into the broth and bring to a boil. This boiling broth is what you use when you can the poultry.

For other types of meat, take any large bones and crack them open. Add them to a pot full of water and cook on medium heat for up to 4 hours. Remove any meat remaining on the bones and put the meat into the broth. Bring to a boil. The broth is now ready to be used for canning.

POULTRY

When you can poultry, dress your chicken and chill it for at least 6 hours. Cut the bird up into the size of pieces you want to can and trim off any excess fat.

Poultry can be raw packed, meaning you fill the canning jars with just the meat and a teaspoon of salt. If you use this method, leave 1 1/2 inches of headspace in each jar.

You can also hot pack your poultry. When you use this method, you cook the poultry until its 2/3rd cooked, then pack it in the canning jars. Pour boiling broth over the meat and leave an inch and a half of head space.

Pint-sized jars of poultry should be processed in a dial-gauge canner for an hour and 15 minutes if the bones have been removed, and an hour and 5 minutes if the bones have been left in. Adjust pressure as needed based on the chart above, if you live above sea level.

MEATS

Meat should be chilled and fresh. Remove any big bones and trim as much fat from the meat as you can.

If you're canning ground meat or sausage, you need to cook it first until lightly brown. This will help hold the meat together. Ground meat should be canned using meat broth that's been brought to a boil or tomato sauce. Ground meat requires an inch of headspace.

Strips or chunks of meat can also be canned. Wild game should be soaked in a salt brine prior to canning.

You can hot pack meat with boiling broth or tomato juice, or you can raw pack just the meat with no liquid added. An inch of headspace is required for both the raw and hot packing methods.

Pint-sized jars of meat should be processed in a pressure canner for 75 minutes. Use the chart at the appendix to determine the proper pressure to use for the altitude at which you live.

SEAFOOD

A pressure canner can be used to cook all sorts of seafood, including clams, crabs, and fish such as tuna.

CLAMS

Fresh clams are a popular choice for canning. Wash and clean clam meat. Boil it for a couple minutes, then add the meat and boiling water to the canning jars, leaving an inch of headspace.
Pint-sized jars should be processed for an hour.

CRAB

TIP: It isn't recommended that you can crab meat because it will give it an acidic flavor. Freezing crab is the preferable method of storing it. That said, if you want to can crab meat, it can be done. Boil your crab for a half hour in water with a cup of lemon juice and 3 tablespoons of salt added per gallon of water.

Remove the meat from the shell and soak for five minutes in fresh water with lemon juice and added salt. After soaking, gently press the meat to remove as much water as possible.
Fill pint-sized canning jars with the crab meat and add 5 tablespoons of lemon juice to each jar. Be sure to leave an inch of headspace.
Pint-sized jars should be processed for 70 minutes at the pressure indicated in the chart at the appendix section.

FISH

Fish needs to be gutted, scaled and bled immediately after they're caught. Cut off the head, tail and fins. Keep fish cool until you're ready to can them.

TIP: The bones can be left in most fish because they become soft during the canning process. This will add extra calcium to your canned fish. Cut fish into 3-inch strips and pack into canning jars. You can add a teaspoon of salt per pint-sized jar if you want to. You don't need to add any liquid to the fish.

Pint-sized jars should be processed for 100 minutes. Check the chart at the appendix section for the pressure to process it at.

TIP: Be aware; crystals of magnesium ammonium phosphate may form in tuna or salmon during the canning process. These crystals are safe to consume and will dissolve when you cook the fish.

TUNA

Tuna requires special preparation.

It needs to be cooked at 350 degrees F for an hour or steamed for 3 hours. The internal temperature of the tuna needs to reach 175 degrees.

Refrigerate overnight, then skin the cooked fish. Debone the fish, skin it and cut away any discolored sections of meat.

Tuna needs to be hot packed into oil or water. Leave an inch of headspace.

Process for 100 minutes at the pressure indicated in the chart in the appendix section.

HOW TO CAN YOUR FAVORITE HOMEMADE SOUP

Most soups made at home can safely be canned using the pressure canning method.

The following items should not be added to soups you plan on canning:

- Purees
- Rice
- Flour
- Noodles
- Milk or other dairy products
- Thickeners

If the soup recipe you're making calls for any of these items, you can add most of them when you cook the soup after opening the jar to consume it. For soups that need to be pureed, can them chunky and puree them when you plan on eating them.

The following items need to be cooked before you add them to your soup:

- Meat
- Vegetables
- Beans
- Peas

Jars should be filled half full with the solid ingredients, then have boiling broth or soup stock poured over the top. Leave an inch of headspace.

Pints of soup should be processed for an hour. Quarts need to be processed for an hour and 20 minutes. Use the chart in the meat section to determine how to adjust pressure based on your altitude. Soups with seafood in them should be processed for an additional 40 minutes.

24. Tomato Soup

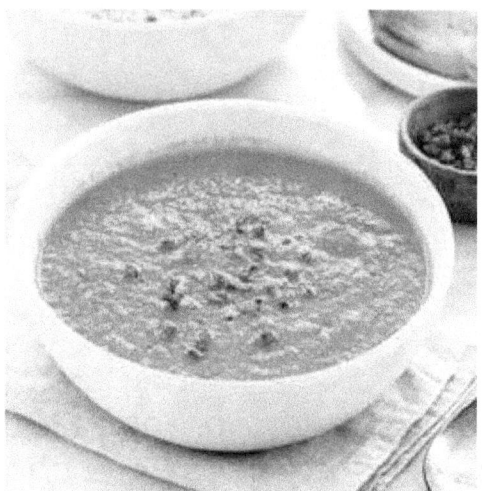

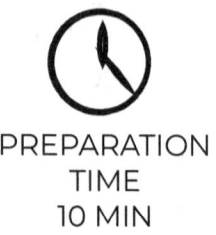

PREPARATION TIME
10 MIN

COOK TIME
2 HOURS

SERVING
8

INGREDIENTS

- 7 lbs. tomatoes, diced
- ½ Tsp. black pepper
- 1 Tsp. celery seed
- 2 Tsp. garlic, minced
- 2 Bay leaves
- 2 Tsp. dried basil
- 1 Tbsp. dried oregano
- 3 Tbsp. brown sugar
- 3 Tbsp. tomato paste
- ½ Cup water
- 1 Cup onion, diced
- 1 ½ Tsp. salt

DIRECTIONS

1. Add onion and tomatoes in a large pot along with ½ cup water, and cook for 30 minutes.
2. Remove pot from heat and puree the tomatoes using a blender until smooth.
3. Return the tomato puree pot on the heat. Add spices, herbs, sugar, and tomato paste. Stir well and bring to simmer for 60 minutes. Adjust salt.
4. Remove pot from heat. Add 1 tablespoon of lemon juice to each jar.
5. Fill a jar with soup. Leave ½ an inch headspace.
6. Seal jars with lids and process in a boiling water bath for 40 minutes.
7. Remove jars from the water bath and let it cool completely.
8. Check seals of jars. Label and store.

Nutritions: Calories: 99 Cal; Protein: 4 g; Sugar: 15 g; Fat: 1 g; Carbs: 22 g

25. Canned Mushroom Soup

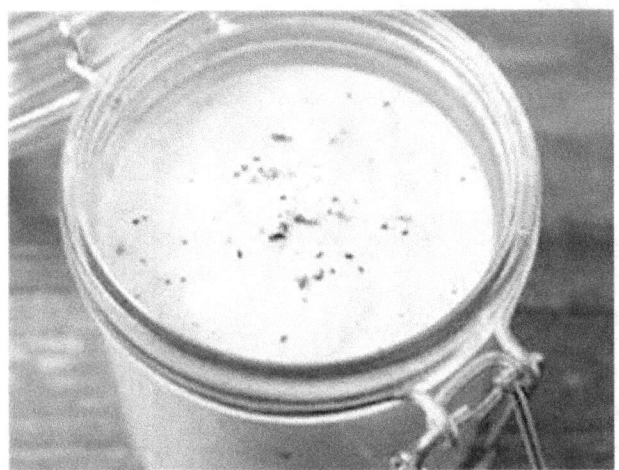

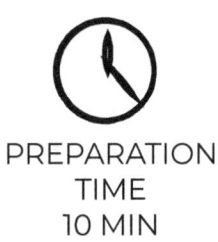

PREPARATION TIME
10 MIN

COOK TIME
2 H 20

SERVING
12

INGREDIENTS

- 6 Cups baby Bella mushrooms, sliced
- 16 Cups milk
- 2 Cups tapioca starch
- 1 Cup butter
- 4 Tbsp. sea salt

DIRECTIONS

1. Melt butter in a large saucepan over medium heat.
2. Add mushrooms and sauté for 5 minutes.
3. Add tapioca starch and salt and stir well. Slowly add milk and stir well.
4. Stir well and cook over medium heat until thickened.
5. Remove pan from heat. Ladle soup into the clean jars. Leave 1/2 an inch headspace.
6. Seal jars with lids and process in a boiling water bath for 2 hours.
7. Remove jars from the water bath and let it cool completely.
8. Check seals of jars. Label and store.

Nutritions: Calories: 536 Cal; Protein: 12.1 g; Sugar: 16.3 g; Fat: 37.5 g; Carbs: 40.7 g

26. Celery Soup

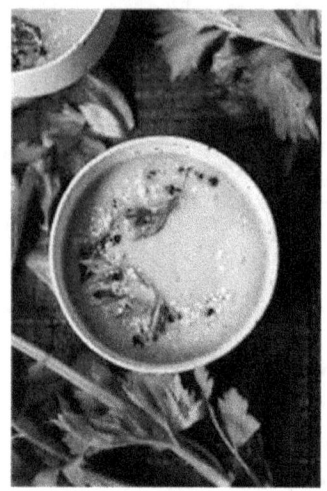

PREPARATION TIME
10 MIN

COOK TIME
30 MIN

SERVING
20

INGREDIENTS

- 1 lb. Celery, diced
- 1 Onion, diced
- 4 Cups vegetable stock
- 1 Medium potato, peeled and diced
- 1 Tbsp. olive oil
- 1 Garlic clove, minced
- ½ Cup dry white wine

DIRECTIONS

1. Heat oil in a large pot over medium heat. Add onions, garlic, and celery and sauté until translucent, about 10 minutes. Add wine and stir well.
2. Add potatoes, stock, pepper, and salt, and simmer for 5 minutes.
3. Remove the pot from the heat.
4. Add lids and rings. Place the jar into the pressure canner.
5. Process can soup for 10 minutes at 11 lbs. pressure in a pressure canner.
6. Once done, cool canner, remove the lid and let the jars stand for 10 minutes before removing from canner.
7. Remove carrot jars from the canner and place them on the counter for 1-2 hours.
8. Check the seals of jars. Label and store.

Nutritions: Calories: 27 Cal; Protein: 0.5 g; Sugar: 1.1 g; Fat: 1.2 g; Carbs: 3.7 g

27. Navy Bean Soup

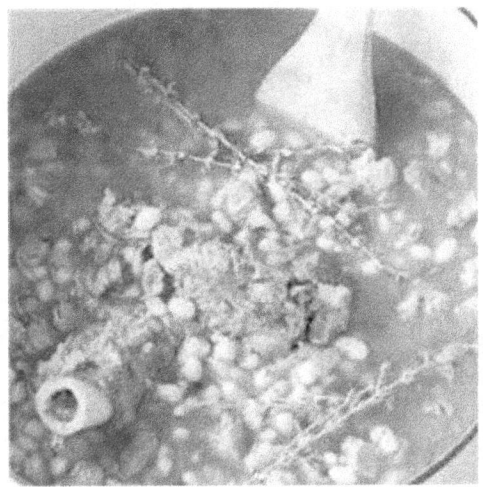

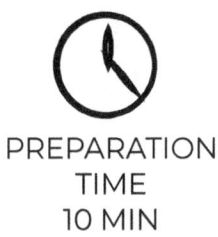

PREPARATION TIME
10 MIN

COOK TIME
1 H 40

SERVING
12

INGREDIENTS

- 1 Cup dried navy beans
- 1 1/2 Cups carrot, sliced
- 3 Cups ham, diced
- 4 Cups chicken broth

DIRECTIONS

1. Add beans into the large bowl and cover with water. Cover it and let it sit overnight.
2. Drain beans well. Add beans into the large pot and cover at least 2 inches of water. Bring it to boil, and simmer for 30 minutes.
3. Add broth to the saucepan and bring it to boil.
4. Fill clean jars with an equal amount of carrots, ham, and beans. Top with hot broth. Leave a 1 inch headspace.
5. Add lids and rings. Place the jar into the pressure canner.
6. Process can soup pints for 75 minutes, quarts for 90 minutes at 10 lbs. pressure in a pressure canner.
7. Check the seals of jars. Label and store.

Nutritions: Calories: 130 Cal; Protein: 11 g; Sugar: 2 g; Fat: 11 g; Carbs: 13 g

28. Carrot Soup

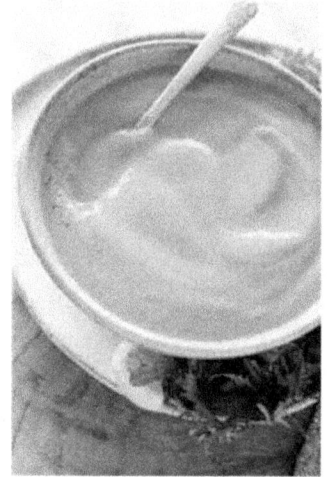

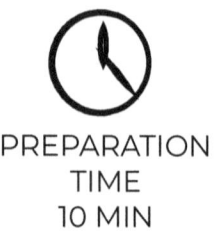

PREPARATION TIME
10 MIN

COOK TIME
1 H 35

SERVING
12

INGREDIENTS

- 4 lbs. Carrots, washed, peeled & sliced
- 1 lb. Fennel bulb, chopped
- 1 Tsp. Dried thyme
- 2 Tsp. Onion powder
- 12 cups Vegetable stock
- 1 Tbsp. Olive oil
- 1/2 Tsp. Ground cumin
- 1 Tsp. Ground black pepper
- 1 Tsp. Ground coriander
- 1 Tsp. Ground ginger
- 2 Tbsp. Salt

DIRECTIONS

1. Heat oil in a saucepan over medium heat.
2. Add fennel and sauté until translucent.
3. Add carrots and 4 cups of stock and let it simmer for 30 minutes.
4. Remove saucepan from heat, and using a blender, puree the carrots until smooth.
5. Return the saucepan on the heat.
6. Add the remaining ingredients and stir well, and cook on low heat for 20-30 minutes.
7. Ladle soup into the clean jars. Leave a 1 inch headspace.
8. Seal the jar with the lids. Process it in a water bath canner for 40 minutes.
9. Remove the jars from the water bath and let it cool completely.
10. Check the seals of jars. Label and store.

Nutritions: Calories: 86 Cal; Protein: 2 g; Sugar: 7 g; Fat: 1 g; Carbs: 18 g

29. Taco Turkey Stew

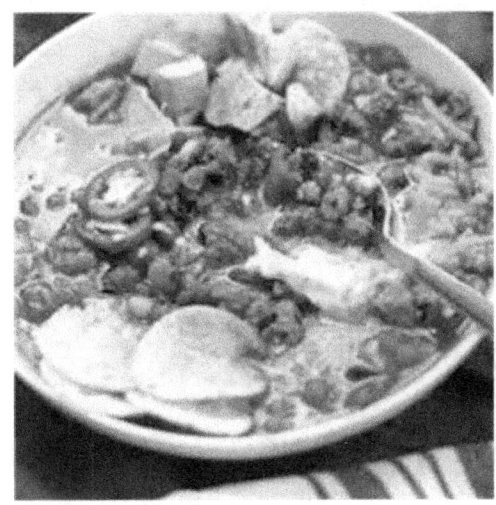

INGREDIENTS

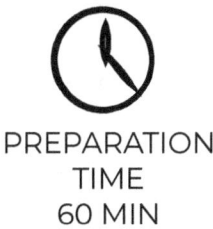

PREPARATION TIME 60 MIN

COOK TIME 8-12 H DEHYDRATION

SERVING 4

- 2 & 1/4 Pounds of turkey mince, lean
- 1 Tbsp. Olive oil
- 2 Chopped bell peppers, red
- 1 Chopped onion, red
- 1 x 14-oz. Can of drained black beans
- 1 x 12-oz. Can of drained sweet corn
- 1 Packet of spice mixture, taco
- 1 x 14-oz. Can of tomatoes, diced
- Salt, kosher, as desired
- 1 Bunch of chopped cilantros, fresh
- 1 Tbsp. Of powdered cheddar cheese, freeze dried
- 1 Handful of crumbled corn chips

DIRECTIONS

1. Heat oil in a large sized pan. Add onions. Cook until golden and softened.
2. Add the turkey. Cook it until it has fully browned. Transfer it to the colander. Drain the turkey. Return to pan.
3. Add corn, beans, red pepper and taco spice blend.
4. Stir occasionally as you continue cooking for five minutes or so.
5. Add diced tomatoes and juice. Bring to boil.
6. Add cilantro. Season as desired.
7. Reduce the heat down to low. Place a lid on the pan. Allow cooking for 15 more minutes.
8. Remove from heat. Allow to thoroughly cool.
9. Spread turkey stew on pre-lined dehydrator trays.
10. Dehydrate at 145 degrees F for eight to 12 hours, until stew is brittle. Allow it to cool.
11. Divide dried meal into equal portions in separate zipper top plastic bags. Store until you are ready to use them.

Nutritions: Calories: 102 Cal; Protein: 0 g; Sodium: 3 g; Fat: 0 g; Carbs: 27 g

30. Bean and Bacon Soup

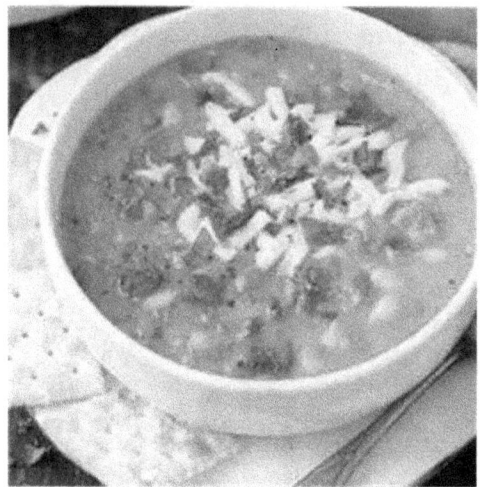

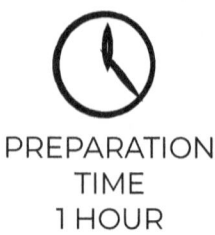

PREPARATION TIME
1 HOUR

COOK TIME
2 HOUR

SERVING
32 CUPS

INGREDIENTS

- 2 Pounds of dried navy beans that have been soaked in water overnight
- 8 Cups of tomato juice
- 8 Cups of chicken or vegetable stock
- 2 Cups of carrots
- 4 Cups of white potatoes, about 6 medium
- 3 Cups of chopped celery, about 6 stalks
- 1 Tablespoon of salt
- 2 Teaspoons of black pepper
- 2 Bay leaves
- 3 Cups of diced onion, about 6 medium
- 2 Pounds of bacon
- Water

DIRECTIONS

1. Slice carrots and celery. Dice onions, potatoes, and bacon.
2. Mix all ingredients except for the bacon and onions in a large stockpot, bring to a boil, and reduce heat to medium. Let it simmer.
3. Fry bacon in a large skillet over medium heat until golden browned, about 10 minutes. Add the onions. Sauté for an additional 10 minutes.
4. Add bacon and onions to the bean mixture. If the soup seems too thick, add some water until you get the preferred consistency. Heat it until it simmers, about 30-35 more minutes.
5. Remove bay leaves with tongs, and pour equal amounts of the soup into jars.
6. Pressure cook for 1 hour at 10 pounds for the weighted gauge of the pressure canner, or 11 pounds if the pressure canner has a dial gauge.
7. Remove the jars, and let them cool completely at room temperature before storing. This can take about a day.

Nutritions: Calories: 590 Cal; Protein: 29.65 g; Fiber: 14.2 g; Fat: 36.95 g; Carbs: 45.34 g

31. Mexican Turkey Soup

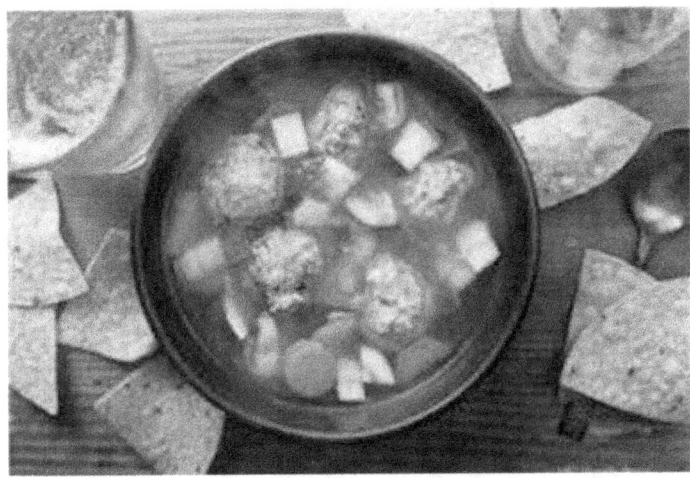

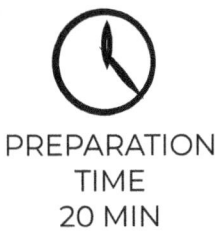

PREPARATION TIME
20 MIN

COOK TIME
1 H 30

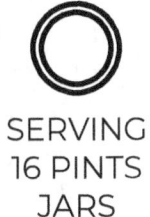

SERVING
16 PINTS JARS

INGREDIENTS

- 6 Cups of cooked turkey, chopped
- 2 Cups of chopped onions
- 8 Ounces can of Mexican green chilies, chopped and drained
- ¼ Cup of taco seasoning mix, packed
- 28 Ounces of crushed tomatoes with the juices
- 16 Cups of turkey or chicken broth
- 3 Cups of corn
- 1 ½ Tablespoons of extra virgin olive oil

DIRECTIONS

1. In a large stockpot, warm olive oil on medium-high heat. Sauté the onions until tender and fragrant, about 2 minutes on medium-high heat. Reduce heat to medium-low.
2. Add taco seasoning and the chilies. Cook and stir for another 3 minutes, add in the tomatoes and the broth. Bring to a boil, and then add the corn and the turkey.
3. Reduce heat to low, and let it simmer for 10 minutes.
4. Ladle it equally into the jars.
5. Process pints at 10 pounds for 75 minutes and quarts at 10 pounds for 90 minutes for the weighted gauge of the pressure canner, or 11 pounds if the pressure canner has a dial gauge.
6. Remove jars, and let cool until it is at room temperature. This may take about a day.

Nutritions: Calories: 580 Cal; Protein: 63.66 g; Fiber: 3.2 g; Fat: 76.84 g; Carbs: 30.08 g

32. Vegetarian Vegetable Soup

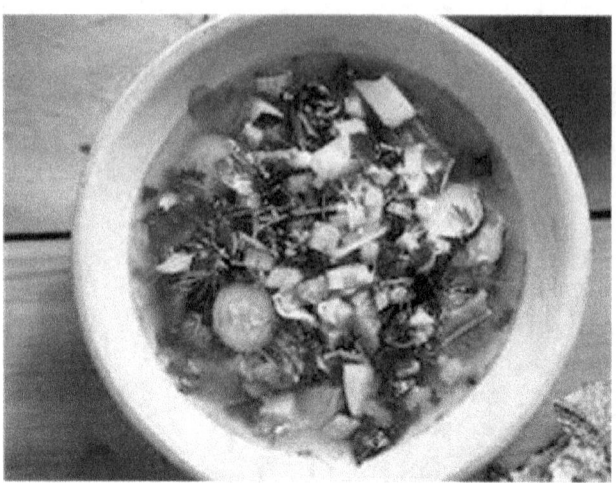

INGREDIENTS

- 1 Cup chopped onion
- 1 Cup chopped celery
- 1 Cup diced potatoes
- 2 Pounds boneless chicken breasts
- 2 Teaspoons salt
- 2 Teaspoons poultry seasoning
- 4 Tablespoons white wine
- Enough chicken stock to fill the jars

PREPARATION TIME
3 HOURS

COOK TIME
3 HOURS

SERVING
9 QUART JARS

DIRECTIONS

1. In a large stock pot, heat the olive oil on medium-high heat. Sauté leeks and onions until tender and fragrant, about 8-10 minutes.
2. Add the remaining ingredients, and bring to a boil. Reduce the heat to medium-low, and let it simmer gently for about an hour until all the vegetables are tender. Season to taste with kosher salt and freshly ground pepper.
3. Pour the soup equally into jars.
4. Process for 90 minutes at 10 pounds of pressure for the weighted gauge of the pressure canner, or 11 pounds if the pressure canner has a dial gauge.
5. Remove the jars, and let them cool until it is at room temperature. This may take about a day.

Nutritions: Calories: 322 Cal; Protein: 8.07 g; Fiber: 11.3 g; Fat: 7.57 g; Carbs: 59.52 g

33. Canned Vegetable Soup

This pressure canned soup tastes amazing. It is a healthy recipe as tomatoes are a good source of potassium, which is an essential mineral for heart disease prevention and blood pressure control. You will enjoy it.

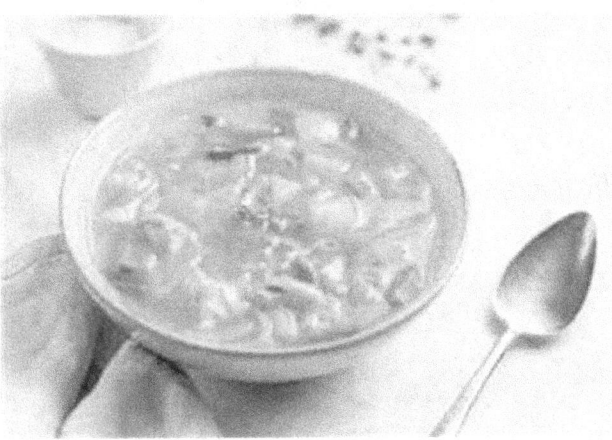

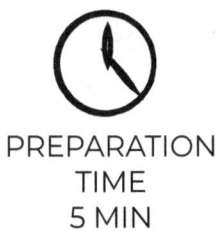

PREPARATION TIME
5 MIN

COOK TIME
30 MIN

SERVING
7

INGREDIENTS

- 8 Cups chopped tomatoes, peeled and cored
- 6 Cups cubed potatoes, peeled
- 6 Cups carrots, 3/4 inch slices
- 4 Cups green lima beans
- 4 Cups corn kernels, uncooked
- 2 Cups celery, 1-inch slices
- 2 Cups onions, chopped
- 6 Cups water
- Optional: Salt and pepper to taste

DIRECTIONS

1. Combine vegetables in a large saucepot, and then add water.
2. Bring to boil for about 25 minutes on high, then reduce heat to low and simmer for about 5 minutes.
3. Now season with pepper and salt if desired.
4. Scoop the hot soup into hot quart jars. Make sure you leave a 1 inch headspace.
5. If needed, remove air bubbles adjusting the headspace. Wipe the rims of the jars using a clean damp towel.
6. Place the lids and process quart jars in a pressure canner for about 85 minutes at 11 pounds pressure if using a dial-gauge canner, or a 10 pounds pressure if using a weighted-gauge canner.

Nutritions: Calories: 354 Cal; Carbs: 75.1g; Protein: 14.1g; Sugar: 17.1g; Fiber 15.4g

34. Pressure Canned Chicken Soup

This is truly and honestly the best way to preserve chicken soup. The soup is full of flavor, delicious, and perfect that all your family members will love.

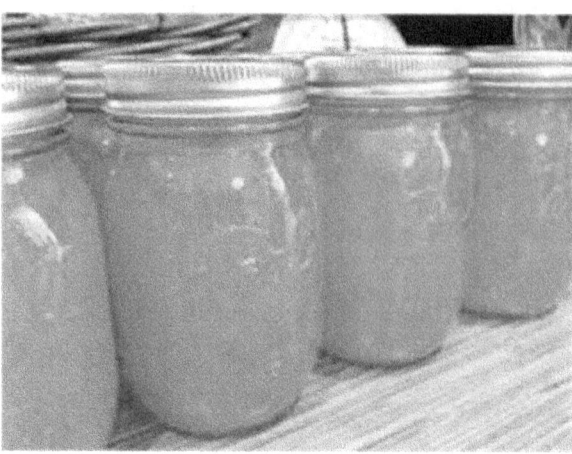

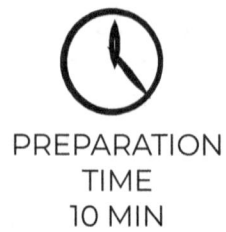

PREPARATION TIME
10 MIN

COOK TIME
1 HOUR

INGREDIENTS

- 16 Cups Chicken stock
- 1-1/2 Cups celery, diced
- 3 Cups chicken, diced
- 1 Cup onion, diced
- 1-1/2 Cups carrots, sliced
- Optional: 3 Chicken bouillon cubes
- Optional: Salt and pepper to taste

SERVING
4

DIRECTIONS

1. Combine chicken stock, celery, chicken, onion, and carrots in a large saucepot, and bring it to boil on high, for about 30 minutes.
2. Reduce the heat to medium-low and simmer for about 30 minutes.
3. Add the optional ingredients and cook until bouillon cubes dissolve if desired.
4. Scoop the hot soup into hot quart jars and leave a 1 inch headspace.
5. If needed, remove air bubbles, adjusting headspace. Wipe the rims of the jars using a clean damp paper towel.
6. Now apply the 2-piece metal caps.
7. Process quart jars in a pressure canner for 90 minutes at 11 pounds pressure if using a dial-gauge canner, or a 10 pounds pressure if using a weighted-gauge canner.

Nutritions: Calories: 293 Cal, Carbs: 24.6g; Protein 35.7g; Sugar: 13.4g; Fiber: 6.6g

35. Canned Carrot and Ginger Soup

This pressure canned soup has a unique sweetness. It is also a healthy recipe as carrots are linked to a reduced risk of heart disease and improved eye health. Everyone will be left yearning for more.

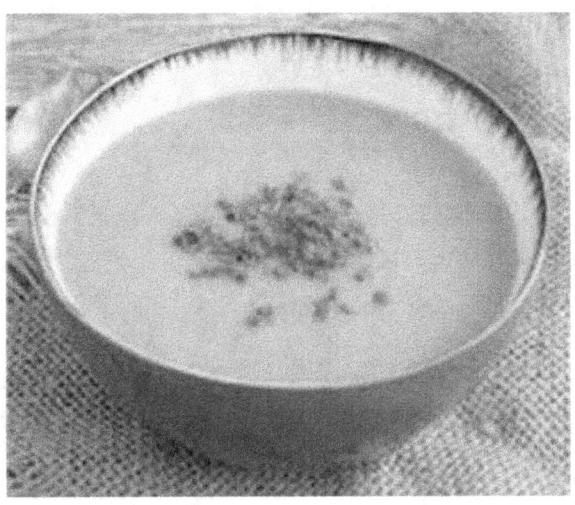

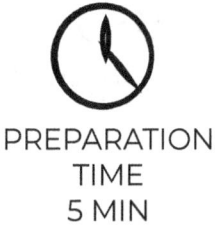
PREPARATION TIME
5 MIN

COOK TIME
1 HOUR

SERVING
7

INGREDIENTS

- 3 Tbsp. butter
- 1 Large peeled Spanish onion, diced
- 2 Garlic cloves, whole and peeled
- 3 lbs. Peeled and sliced carrots
- 2 Sliced ribs celery
- 3 Tbsp. fresh ginger, peeled and chopped
- 8 Cups vegetable or chicken stock
- 1 Tbsp. coriander, ground
- 1/2 Cup honey
- Salt and black pepper to taste

DIRECTIONS

1. Melt butter in a stockpot, stainless steel, over high-medium heat.
2. Add onion, garlic, carrots, celery, and ginger and sauté for about 10 minutes. Stir frequently.
3. Add stock and bring to a boil. Reduce the heat and simmer for 30-35 minutes until carrots are tender.
4. Remove from the heat, then add ginger, coriander, and honey.
5. Pour the soup into an immersion blender and blend until smooth.
6. Scoop the hot soup into sterilized jars and leave a 1 inch headspace.
7. If needed, remove air bubbles adjusting headspace. Wipe the rims of the jars using a clean damp paper towel.
8. Now apply the 2-piece metal caps.
9. Process quart jars in a pressure canner for 85 minutes at 11 pounds pressure if using a dial-gauge canner, or a 10 pounds pressure if using a weighted-gauge canner.

Nutritions: Calories: 224 Cal; Carbs 43.5g; Protein: 3g; Sugar: 31.1g; Fiber 5.6g

36. Pressure Canned Tomato Soup

This is one of the best pressure canned recipes to prepare in your home. This tomato soup may probably become your family's favorite soup and I bet everyone will enjoy it.

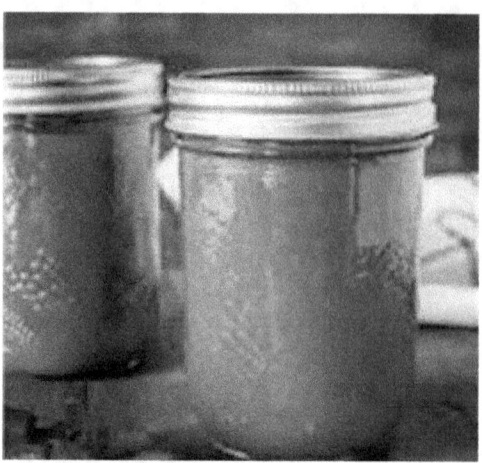

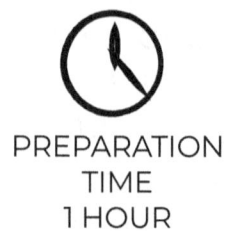

PREPARATION TIME
1 HOUR

COOK TIME
15 MIN

SERVING
20

INGREDIENTS

- 20lbs Rinsed tomatoes, cut into small chunks
- 10 Tbsp. divided lemon juice

DIRECTIONS

1. Place tomatoes in a pot of boiling water, then parboil the tomatoes for about 1-2 minutes until the skins begin to come off.
2. Place a strainer into a large bowl.
3. Now remove and place the tomatoes on the strainer. Run them through a food mill to get rid of skins and seeds.
4. Transfer the puree into a stockpot over low heat and keep it warm until ready to pressure can.
5. Funnel lemon juice and warm tomato puree into canning jars. Leave a 1 inch headspace.
6. If needed, remove air bubbles adjusting headspace. Wipe the rims of the jars using a clean damp paper towel.
7. Now apply the 2-piece metal caps.
8. Process quart jars in a pressure canner for 15 minutes at 11 pounds pressure if using a dial-gauge canner, or 10 pounds pressure if using a weighted-gauge canner.

Nutritions: Calories: 83 Cal; Fat: 0g; Carbs: 13g; Protein: 4g; Sugar: 12g

37. Canned Chicken Stock

This is a stock recipe that you and your family can have all week long without any complaining. It is a comforting, nourishing, and a healthy pressure canned stock.

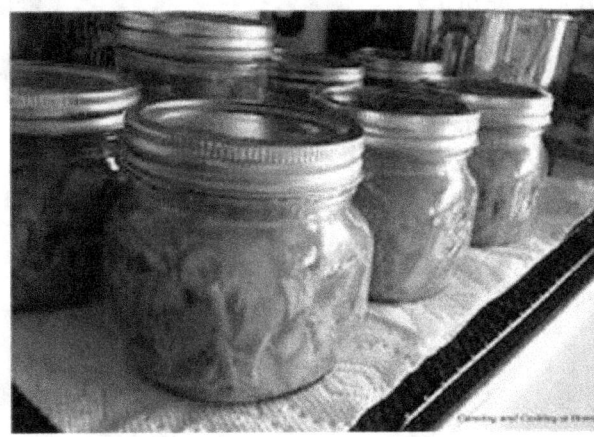

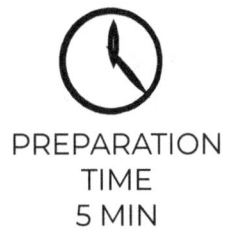

PREPARATION TIME
5 MIN

COOK TIME
2 H 20

SERVING
4

INGREDIENTS

- 16 Cups water
- 3-4 lbs. chicken, pieces cut
- 2 Stalks celery
- 2 Quartered onions, medium
- 1 Tbsp. salt
- 10 Peppercorns

DIRECTIONS

1. Prepare your pressure canner and heat your jars with simmering water. Wash the lids with soapy warm water, and set the bands aside.
2. Place the water and chicken in a large saucepan, then bring it to boil.
3. Reduce the heat and simmer for about 2 hours until the chicken becomes tender. Now remove from the heat and skim off the foam.
4. Remove and reserve the chicken for other use.
5. Meanwhile, strain the stock through several cheesecloth layers or a sieve, and allow it to cool for the fat to solidify. Now skim the fat off.
6. Heat to boil the stock and scoop hot stock into hot pint jars. Leave a 1 inch headspace.
7. Wipe the rims of the jars using a clean damp paper towel.
8. Center the lid on jars, then apply band adjusting until it is a fingertip tight fit.
9. Process the pint jars in a pressure canner for 20 minutes at 11 pounds pressure if using a dial-gauge canner, or 10 pounds pressure if using a weighted-gauge canner.

Nutritions: Calories: 709 Cal; Fat: 13.8g; Carbs: 5.6g; Protein: 132.2g; Sugar: 2.4g

38. American Chicken Stock

Looking for a super delicious stock? American chicken stock is the recipe you are looking for as it is delicious each and every time.

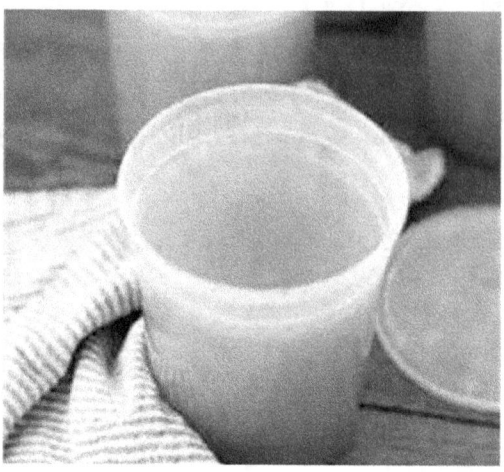

PREPARATION TIME
1 H

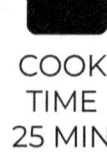

COOK TIME
25 MIN

SERVING
1

INGREDIENTS

- Chicken bones, meat removed
- Water to cover

DIRECTIONS

1. Place bones in a pressure cooker and add water to cover
2. Cook on high pressure for about 30 minutes until the remaining meat falls off from the bones.
3. Strain the stock into a large bowl, then discard the loosened meat from bones. Refrigerate the stock overnight.
4. Skim off and discard the fat, then reheat the stock in a saucepot.
5. Pour the stock into 1 liter US quart jars, leaving a 1 inch headspace. Wipe the rims of the jars using a paper towel, dampened clean.
6. Apply the 2-piece metal caps.
7. Process quart jars in a pressure canner for 25 minutes at 11 pounds pressure if using a dial-gauge canner, or 10 pounds pressure if using a weighted-gauge canner.

Nutritions: Calories: 17 Cal; Fat: 0g; Carbs: 2g; Protein: 2g; Sugar: 2g; Fiber 0g

39. Home-Canned Beef Stock

This makes a healthy beef stock by pressure canning. Pressure canned beef stock is the best option for preparing stock for your family. Beef makes the stock delicious.

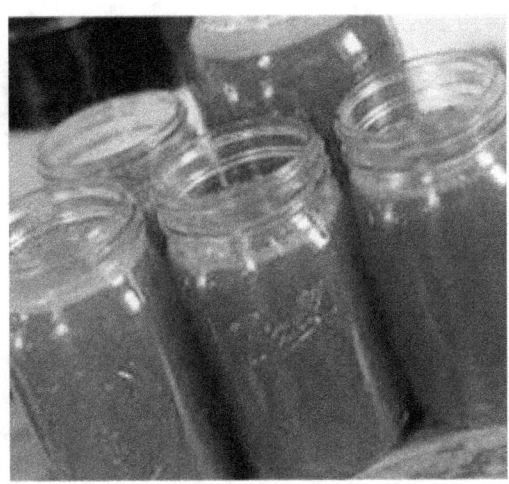

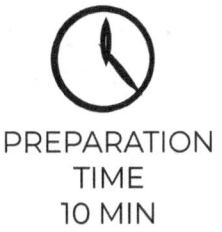

PREPARATION TIME
10 MIN

COOK TIME
2-4 H

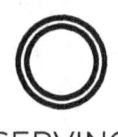

SERVING
4

INGREDIENTS

- 4 lbs. Meaty beef bones
- 1 Finely chopped onion, medium
- 1 Sliced large carrot
- 1 Sliced stalk celery
- 1 Bay leaf, medium
- Salt to taste
- 3 Parsley sprigs, fresh
- 3 Whole peppercorns
- 1 Whole garlic clove
- 1/2 Tbsp. thyme, dried
- 2 Quarts water

DIRECTIONS

1. Optional: Place bones on a large roasting pan, and bake for about 30 minutes. Add the vegetables, then bake them for another 30 minutes until they look like evenly browned bones. Turn occasionally.
2. Transfer the vegetables and bones into a stockpot, scrape the roasting pan with 2 cups water then add it to the stockpot.
3. Add the remaining water, and boil on high heat. Reduce heat to low-medium, skimming off foam.
4. Add bay leaf, cover, and simmer for about 2-4 hours.
5. Remove and discard bones, then strain the stock through a fine sieve.
6. Discard the bay leaf and vegetables, cool, and skim off the fat. It's recommended to refrigerate it overnight.
7. Now bring the stock to boiling and scoop hot stock into hot pint jars. Leave a 1 inch headspace.
8. Wipe the jar rims using a clean damp paper towel, then apply the 2-piece metal caps.
9. Process the quart jars in a pressure canner for 20 minutes at 11 pounds pressure if using a dial-gauge canner, or a 10 pounds pressure if using a weighted-gauge canner.

Nutritions: Calories: 388 Cal; Fat: 28.4g; Carbs: 5.4g; Protein: 26.5g; Sugar: 2.2g

40. Canned Turkey Stock

Do you need to impress your family? It is a perfect and excellent stock recipe that is pressure canned and it is a healthy recipe. You will love it.

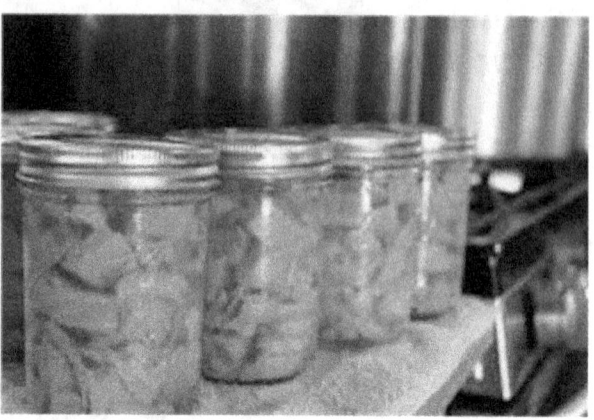

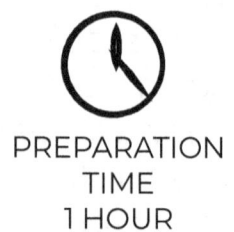

PREPARATION TIME
1 HOUR

COOK TIME
25 MIN

SERVING
1

INGREDIENTS

- Turkey bones, meat removed
- Water to cover
- Optional: salt to taste
- 1 Bay leaf

DIRECTIONS

1. Place the bones and water as such, to cover the bones in a pressure cooker.
2. Add the bay leaf and cook on high pressure for about 30 minutes until the remaining meat falls off from the bones.
3. Strain the stock into a large bowl, and then discard loosened meat from bones. Refrigerate the stock overnight.
4. Skim off and discard the fat, and then reheat the stock in a saucepot.
5. Pour the stock into quart jars leaving a 1 inch headspace. Wipe the rims of the jars using a clean damp paper towel.
6. Apply the 2-piece metal caps.
7. Process the quart jars in a pressure canner for 25 minutes at 11 pounds pressure if using a dial-gauge canner, or a 10 pounds pressure if using a weighted-gauge canner.

Nutritions: Calories: 20 Cal; Fat: 0g; Carbs: 1g; Protein: 4g; Sugar: 1g; Fiber 0g

41. Pressure Canned Turkey Broth

This is a fancy way to prepare and serve turkey broth, impressing all your guests and your kids. This pressure canned turkey broth is a recipe as such that everyone might be left yearning for more.

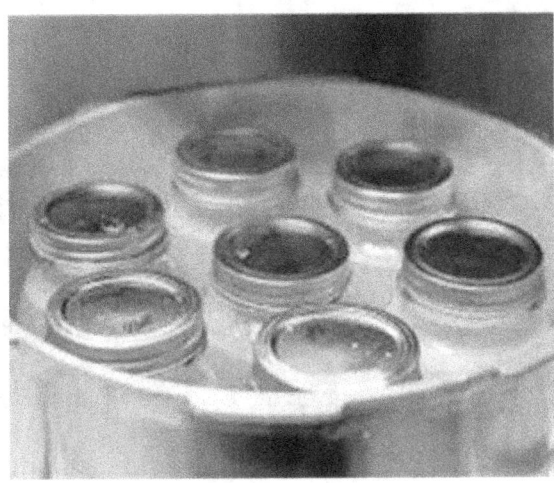

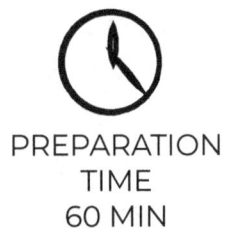

PREPARATION TIME
60 MIN

COOK TIME
30-45 MIN

SERVING
2

INGREDIENTS

- Turkey carcass bones, meat removed
- Optional: 2 quartered onions
- Optional: 2 sliced celery stalks
- Optional: 2 bay leaves
- Optional: Salt to taste
- Water to cover

DIRECTIONS

1. Place the turkey bones and all optional ingredients in a large stockpot, and then add water to cover everything.
2. Cover the pot and simmer for about 30-45 minutes until the remaining meat tidbits fall off easily.
3. Remove and discard the bones, then strain the broth and discard bay leaves and vegetables.
4. Cool the broth, then skim off the fat and discard it. Season with salt if desired.
5. Reheat your broth to boiling.
6. Scoop broth into quart jars. Leave a 1 inch headspace.
7. Wipe the jar rims using a clean damp paper towel, and then apply the 2-piece metal caps.
8. Process the quart jars in a pressure canner for 25 minutes at 11 pounds pressure if using a dial-gauge canner, or a 10 pounds pressure if using a weighted-gauge canner.

Nutritions: Calories: 233 Cal; Fat: 13.1g; Carbs: 12.1g; Protein: 16.5g; Sugar: 4.9g

42. Canned Beef Broth

This recipe is easy, delicious, and quick to cook. Beef broth is a perfect recipe for someone who hates chaos or rushing to get meals ready. Pressure-can beef broth and you won't regret.

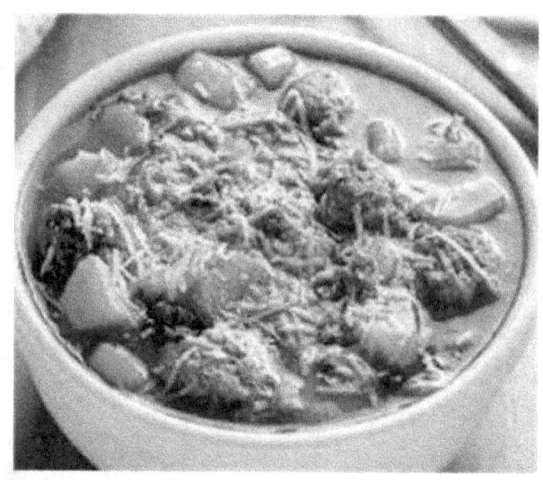

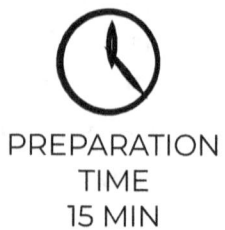

PREPARATION TIME
15 MIN

COOK TIME
3-4 H

SERVING
4

INGREDIENTS

- Optional: 2 quartered onions
- Optional: 2 sliced carrots
- Optional: 2 sliced celery stalks
- Optional: 2 bay leaves
- Salt to taste
- Water to cover

DIRECTIONS

1. Prepare the bones by cracking them to enhance flavor extraction. Now rinse them.
2. Now place the bones and optional ingredients, if using in a large stockpot.
3. Add water to cover everything then cover the pot. Simmer for about 3-4 hours.
4. Remove and discard the bones, vegetables, and bay leaves. Now cool the broth, skim off the fat and discard it.
5. If desired, season with salt.
6. Reheat your broth to boiling.
7. Scoop the hot broth into hot quart jars leaving a 1 inch headspace.
8. Wipe the jar rims using a clean and damp paper towel, and then apply the 2-piece metal caps.
9. Process the quart jars in a pressure canner for 25 minutes at 11 pounds pressure if using a dial-gauge canner, or a 10 pounds pressure if using a weighted-gauge canner.

Nutritions: Calories: 207 Cal; Fat: 7.8g; Fat: 2.9g; Carbs: 9.1g; Protein: 24.3g; Sugar: 3.9g

43. Pressure Canned Chicken Broth

This chicken broth is fast, easy to make, juicy, and delicious. It is a recipe that is best prepared by pressure canning, and will make you feel confident in using a pressure canner.

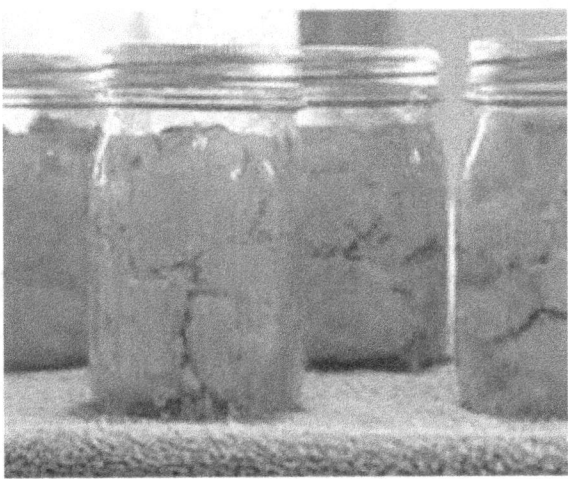

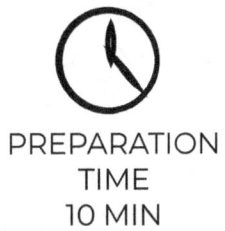

PREPARATION TIME
10 MIN

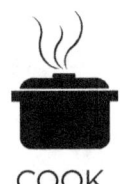

COOK TIME
30-45 MIN

SERVING
2

INGREDIENTS

- Chicken carcass bones, meat removed
- Optional: 2 quartered onions
- Optional: 2 sliced celery stalks
- Optional: 2 bay leaves
- Optional: Salt to taste
- Water to cover

DIRECTIONS

1. Place the chicken bones and all optional ingredients in a stockpot, large, then add water to cover everything.
2. Cover the pot and simmer for about 30-45 minutes until the remaining meat tidbits fall off easily.
3. Remove and discard the bones, then strain the broth and discard bay leaves and vegetables.
4. Cool the broth, then skim off the fat and discard it. Season with salt if desired.
5. Reheat your broth to boiling.
6. Scoop broth into quart jars. Leave a 1 inch headspace.
7. Wipe the jar rims using a clean damp paper towel, then apply the 2-piece metal caps.
8. Process the quart jars in a pressure canner for 25 minutes at 11 pounds pressure if using a dial-gauge canner, or a 10 pounds pressure if using a weighted-gauge canner.

Nutritions: Calories: 233 Cal; Fat: 13.1g; Carbs: 12.1g; Protein: 16.5g; Sugars 4.9g

44. Pressure Canned Beef Stew

Are you looking for an anytime stew recipe to always impress your guests? Pressure canned beef stew is the one for you, as it is delicious and will leave everyone asking for more.

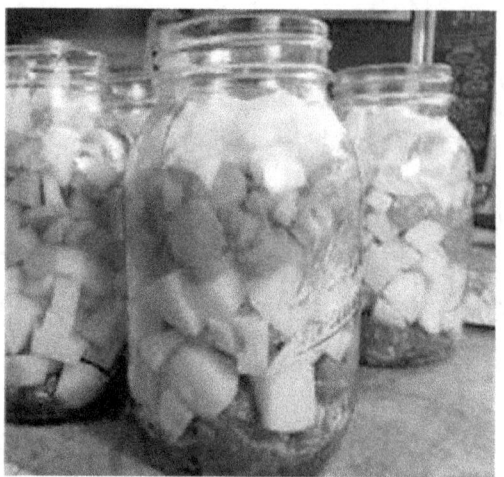

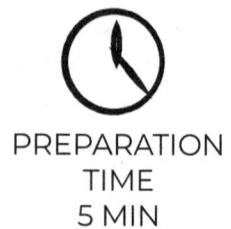
PREPARATION TIME
5 MIN

COOK TIME
30 MIN

SERVING
7

INGREDIENTS

- 4-5lbs Beef stew meat, 1-1/2-inch cubes
- 1 Tbsp. Vegetable oil
- 12 Cups potatoes, peeled and cubed
- 8 Cups carrots, sliced
- 3 Cups celery, chopped
- 3 Cups onion, chopped
- 1 1/2 Tbsp. Salt
- 1 tbsp. Thyme
- 1/2 Tbsp. Pepper
- Water to cover

DIRECTIONS

1. Brown meat in a large saucepot, in oil.
2. Add vegetables and all the seasonings, then cover with water. Boil the stew and remove it from the heat.
3. Scoop the hot stew into hot quart jars. Leave a 1 inch headspace.
4. If needed, remove air bubbles adjusting headspace. Wipe the rims of the jars using a paper towel, dampened clean.
5. Now apply the 2-piece metal caps.
6. Process the quart jars in a pressure canner for about 90 minutes at 11 pounds pressure if using a dial-gauge canner, or a 10 pounds pressure if using a weighted-gauge canner.

Nutritions: Calories: 877 Cal; Fat: 22.6g; Carbs: 59.2g; Protein: 104.6g; Sugars 11.8g

45. Canned Hearty Chili Stew

This is a delicious and a perfect recipe to prepare in a pressure canner. Hearty chili stew is healthy as chilies are linked in the promotion of weight loss.

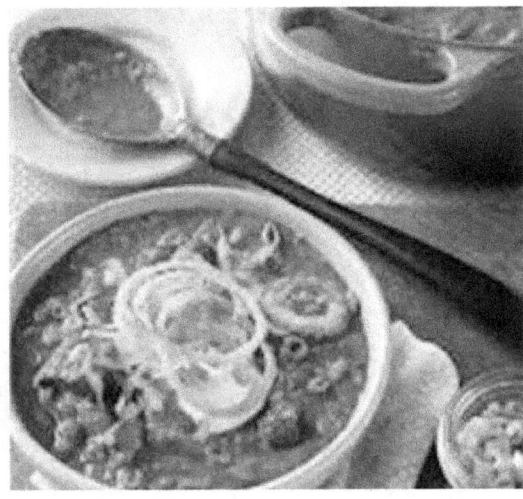

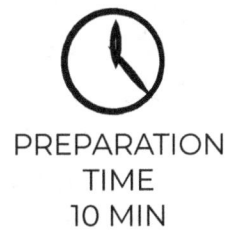

PREPARATION TIME
10 MIN

COOK TIME
1 HOUR

SERVING
6

INGREDIENTS

- 1/4 Cup vegetable oil
- 3 Cups onion, diced
- 2 Minced garlic cloves
- 5 Tbsp. Chili powder
- 2 Tbsp. Cumin seed
- 2 Tbsp. Salt
- 1 Tbsp. Oregano
- 1/2 Tbsp. Pepper
- 1/2 Tbsp. Coriander
- 1/2 Tbsp. Red pepper, crushed
- 6 Cups canned tomatoes, diced and not drained

DIRECTIONS

1. Brown the meat cubes in hot oil lightly, then add garlic and onions. Cook until soft and not brown.
2. Add all the remaining spices and cook for about 5 minutes.
3. Add tomatoes and stir, then bring to a boil on high.
4. Reduce to a medium-low heat and simmer for about 45-60 minutes. Stir occasionally.
5. Scoop hot chili stew into hot pint jars. Leave a 1 inch headspace.
6. If needed, remove the air bubbles, adjusting the headspace. Wipe the rims of the jars using a paper towel, dampened clean.
7. Now apply the 2-piece metal caps.
8. Process the pint jars in a pressure canner for about 90 minutes at 11 pounds pressure if using a dial-gauge canner, or a 10 pounds pressure if using a weighted-gauge canner.

Nutritions: Calories: 733 Cal; Fat: 30g; Carbs: 18.6g; Protein: 95.6g; Sugar: 8.2g; Fiber 6.4g

46. Canned Chili Con Carne

Chili con carne comes with a very wonderful taste when prepared in a pressure canner. It is a delicious stew that you can have any time.

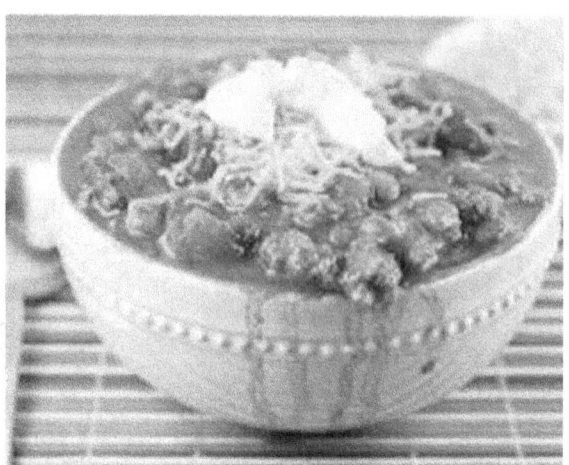

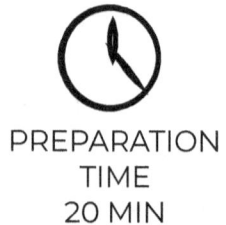

PREPARATION TIME
20 MIN

COOK TIME
1 HOUR

SERVING
9

INGREDIENTS

- 3 Cups pinto bean or red kidney beans, dried and washed
- 5 1/2 Cups water
- 5 Tbsp. Salt, divided
- 3 lbs. Ground beef
- 1 1/2 cups onion, chopped
- 1 Cup pepper, chopped
- 1 Tbsp. Black pepper
- 3-6 Tbsp. Chili powder
- 8 Cups tomatoes, crushed or whole

DIRECTIONS

1. Place the beans in a saucepan, 2-quart, then add cold water to 2-3 inches above beans. Cover and refrigerate for about 12-18 hours to soak. Now drain the beans and discard the water.
2. Place the beans in a saucepot with 5 1/2 cups water. Season with 2 tbsp. salt and bring to a boil for about 25 minutes.
3. Reduce the heat to low and simmer for about 30 minutes.
4. Meanwhile, brown the beef with onions and pepper (optional) in a skillet, then drain the fat off.
5. Add 3 tbsp. salt, and the remaining ingredients together with cooked beans and simmer for about 5 minutes. Make sure not to thicken.
6. Scoop hot chili stew into hot pint jars. Leave a 1 inch headspace. Do not use quart jars.
7. If needed, remove the air bubbles, adjusting the headspace. Wipe the rims of the jars using a clean damp paper towel
8. Now apply the 2-piece metal caps.
9. Process the pint jars in a pressure canner for about 75 minutes at 11 pounds pressure if using a dial-gauge canner, or a 10 pounds pressure if using a weighted-gauge canner.

Nutritions: Calories: 556 Cal; Fat: 11.4g; Carbs 51g; Protein: 61.9g; Sugar: 6.7g

47. Venison Stew with Veggies

This may probably become your favorite pressure canned stew. This venison stew with veggies is an addictive and ultimately delicious recipe that everyone will love.

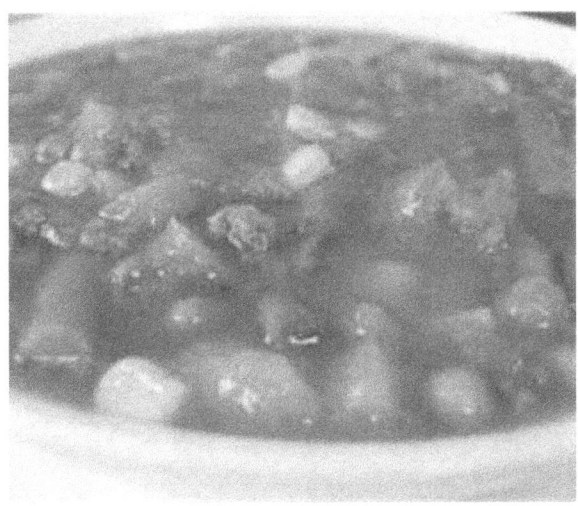

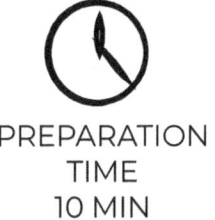
PREPARATION TIME
10 MIN

COOK TIME
30 MIN

SERVING
7

INGREDIENTS

- 1 Tbsp. olive oil
- 4-5 lbs. Trimmed venison stew meat, 1-inch cubes
- 3 Qtrs. Potatoes, 1-inch cubes
- 2 Qtrs. Carrots, largely diced
- 3 Cups celery, chopped
- Optional: 1 1/2 Tbsp. salt
- 1 Tbsp. thyme, dried
- 1/2 - 1 tsp. Black pepper
- Optional: Garlic cloves
- Water to cover

DIRECTIONS

1. Put oil in a large stockpot, and brown the meat cubes.
2. Add veggies and all seasonings, leaving out the thyme and garlic cloves for later use.
3. Pour boiling water to cover the mixture. Boil the mixture fully.
4. Now place thyme and cloves directly into quart jars.
5. Scoop hot venison stew into hot quart jars. Leave a 1 inch headspace.
6. If needed, remove the air bubbles, adjusting the headspace. Wipe the rims of the jars using a clean damp towel
7. Now apply the 2-piece metal caps.
8. Process the pint jars in a pressure canner for about 1 hour 30 minutes at 11 pounds pressure if using a dial-gauge canner, or a 10 pounds pressure if using a weighted-gauge canner.

Nutritions: Calories: 260 Cal; Fat: 4.5g; Carbs: 25g; Protein: 30g; Sugar: 4g; Fiber 3g

Chapter 13.
Full Meal Recipes

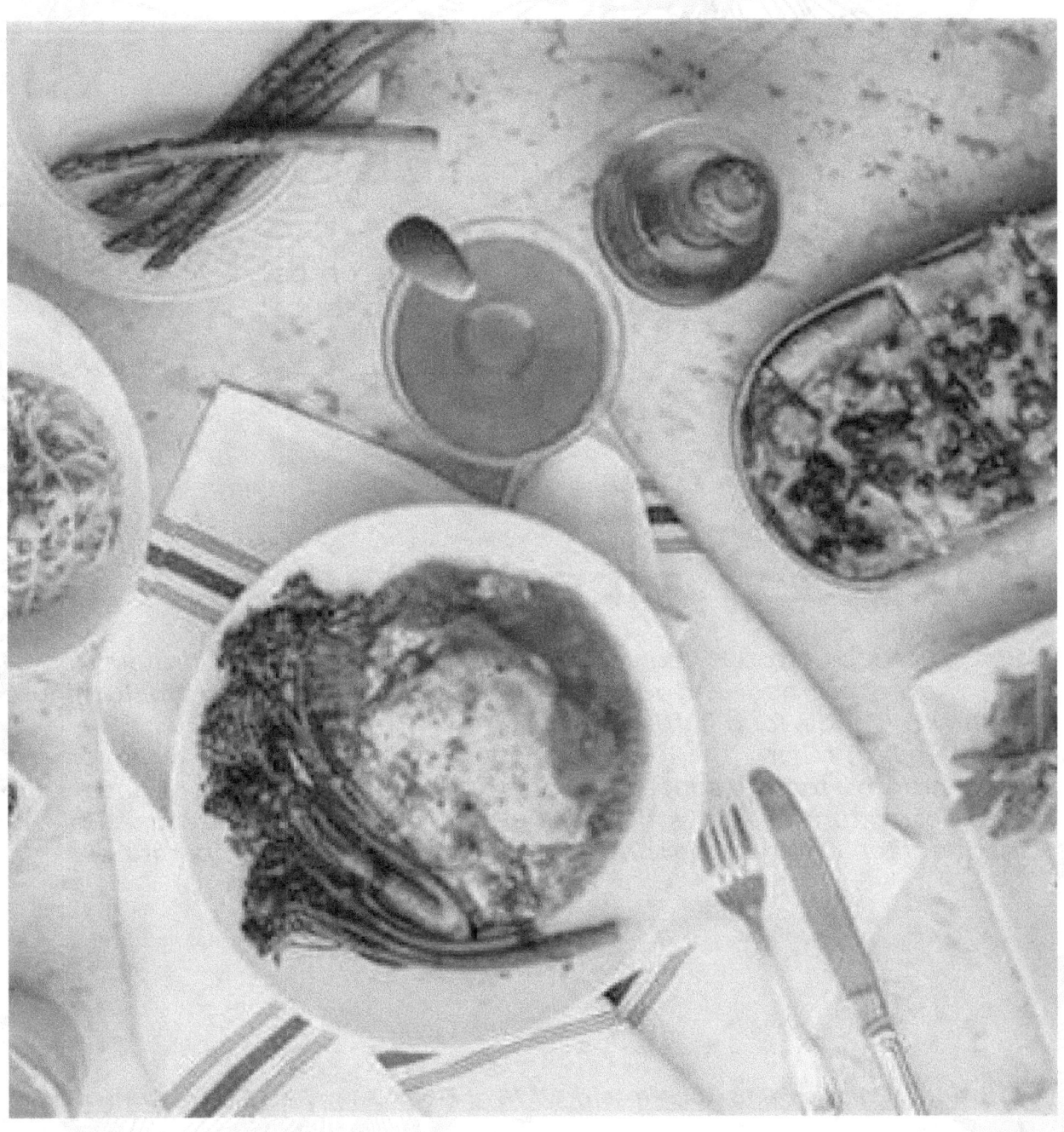

48. Mashed Potatoes and Meatloaf

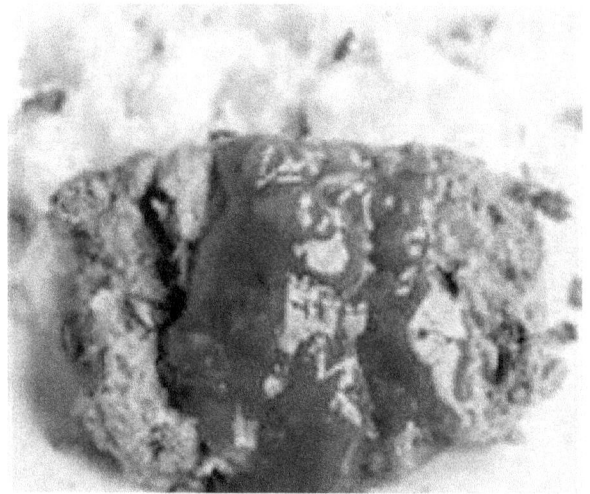

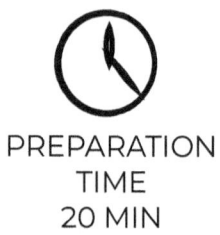

PREPARATION TIME
20 MIN

COOK TIME
50 MIN

SERVING
2

INGREDIENTS

- 2/3 Cup potato flakes
- 2/3 Cup water
- ¼ Cup milk
- 1 Tbsp. butter
- ¼ Tsp. salt
- 1 lb. Ground beef, defrosted
- ½ Cup breadcrumbs
- ¼ Cup tomato sauce
- 1 Egg
- 2 Tbsp. dried herb mix

DIRECTIONS

1. Boil 2/3rd cup of water. Add potato flakes until they are rehydrated. Remove the mixture from heat and add milk, butter, and salt. Let it stand for 10 minutes, then whisk again for a fluffier texture.
2. Meanwhile, preheat the oven to 350F. In a bowl, mash together beef, breadcrumbs, tomato sauce, egg, and dried herbs. Using your hands, shape the beef mixture into a meatloaf and place it in a bread pan to bake. Bake the meatloaf for 30 minutes, or until it reaches safe internal temperatures.

Nutritions: Calories: 698 Cal; Protein: 67.75 g; Fiber: 3.1 g; Fat: 36.9 g; Carbs: 18.66 g

49. Kielbasa and Sauerkraut

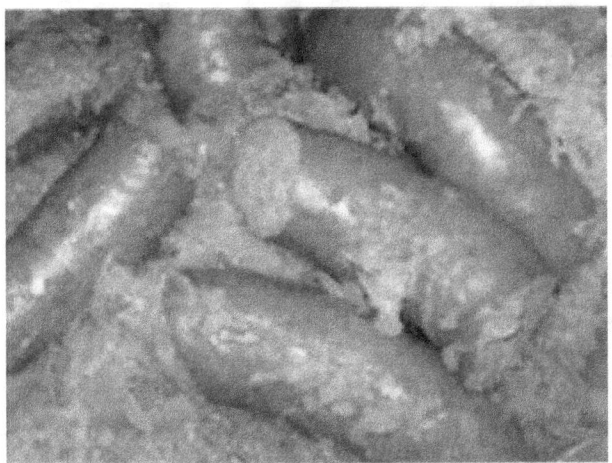

INGREDIENTS

- 3 Potatoes, peeled and diced
- 16 oz. Sauerkraut
- 1lb Kielbasa sausage, cut into ½ inch lengths
- 1 Onion, sliced thin
- ½ Cup butter
- 2 Garlic cloves, minced
- ½ Tsp. Thyme
- ¼ Tsp. Sage
- ¼ Tsp. Black pepper

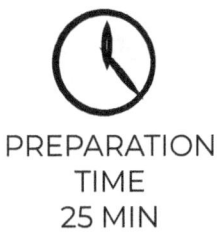

PREPARATION TIME
25 MIN

COOK TIME
3 H 15

SERVING
4

DIRECTIONS

1. Heat cold butter in a pan with the onions. Simmer over medium heat for 10 minutes. Add garlic, thyme, sage, and black pepper. Let it simmer for 2 minutes, so herbs become fragrant.
2. Add sauerkraut with its liquid contents, kielbasa pieces, and potato chunks. Simmer.
3. Pour mixture into a casserole dish and bake at 225 °F for 3 hours.

Nutritions: Calories: 733 Cal; Protein: 28.03 g; Fiber: 12.7 g; Fat: 44.04 g; Carbs: 65.25 g

50. Crockpot Chili

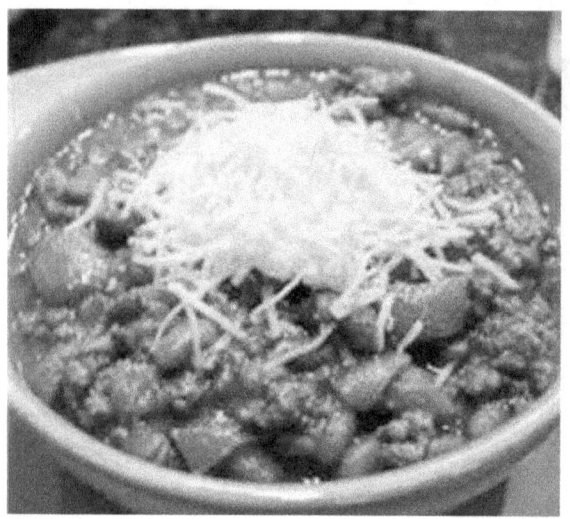

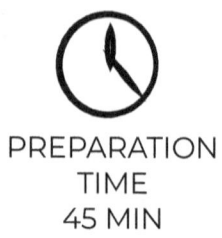

PREPARATION TIME
45 MIN

COOK TIME
3-5 HOUR

SERVING
16

INGREDIENTS

- 1lb Ground beef
- ½ Onion, sliced
- 16 oz. Stewed tomatoes, with juice
- 8 oz. Tomato sauce
- 3 Tbsp. Dried herbs
- 1 Cup dried beans, any mix you like
- 3 Cups soup stock, beef or vegetable

DIRECTIONS

1. Brown your ground beef with 1 tbsp. of your dried herb mix. Add the cooked beef to your crockpot. If you'd like, you can sauté your onion in the retained beef juices. Otherwise, just add them fresh.
2. Combine all of your ingredients in a crockpot and cook over low heat until the beans are cooked all the way through. This takes about 3-5 hours.
3. Consume what you can in two days, freeze the rest in one or two serving increments.

Nutritions: Calories: 77 Cal; Protein: 9.11 g; Fiber: 8 g; Fat: 0.5 g; Carbs: 1.77 g

51. Tuna Sandwiches

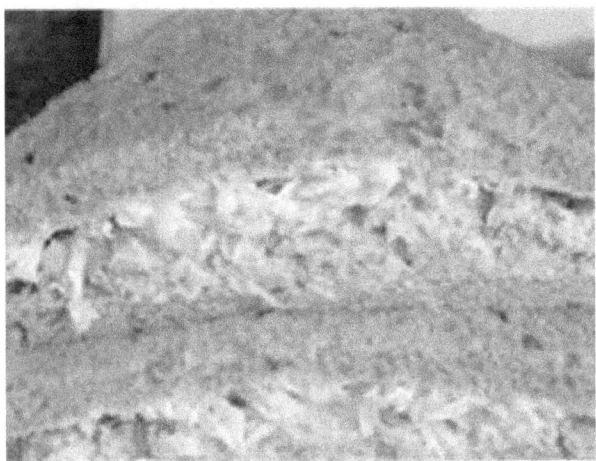

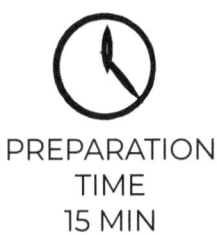

PREPARATION TIME
15 MIN

COOK TIME
1 H 15

SERVING
2

INGREDIENTS

- 1 Jar of tuna in oil
- ¼ Cup mayonnaise
- 3 Cups flour
- 1.5 tbsp. melted butter
- 1.5 Tbsp. sugar
- 1 Tsp. salt
- 1 Tsp. yeast
- 1 Cup whole milk, lukewarm
- ¼ Cup warm water, 115 °F

DIRECTIONS

1. Dissolve one-half tablespoon of the sugar in the warm water and add the yeast. Let it sit for 15 minutes until the yeast becomes frothy.
2. Mix 1.5 cups of flour, the remaining sugar, and salt together. Add the yeast mixture and stir it for about 5 minutes, until no lumps are remaining.
3. Add the remaining flour and knead it for 10 minutes. Let it rest for 15 minutes. Transfer it into a floured bowl and let it rise for 2+ hours. The longer, the better your bread will taste.
4. Punch the dough down, knead it for 5 minutes. Place it in a greased loaf pan and let it rise for 2+ hours. Again, the longer the rise, the better the bread.
5. Bake the bread at 350 °F for 30 minutes, or until the top is golden brown. Remove it from the oven, rub the top with melted butter, and let it rest for half an hour.
6. Drain the tuna, flake it with your fork, and add mayo. Mix it together until you have a wet, sticky tuna salad texture.
7. Slice your bread and place tuna salad on one side of the bread. Top it with another piece and serve!
8. Store leftover bread in saran wrap and tinfoil in the cupboard and eat it within three days for the freshest flavor.

Nutritions: Calories: 994 Cal; Protein: 25.59 g; Fiber: 5.6 g; Fat: 23.79 g; Carbs: 166.35 g

52. Hearty Cowboy Trails Dinner

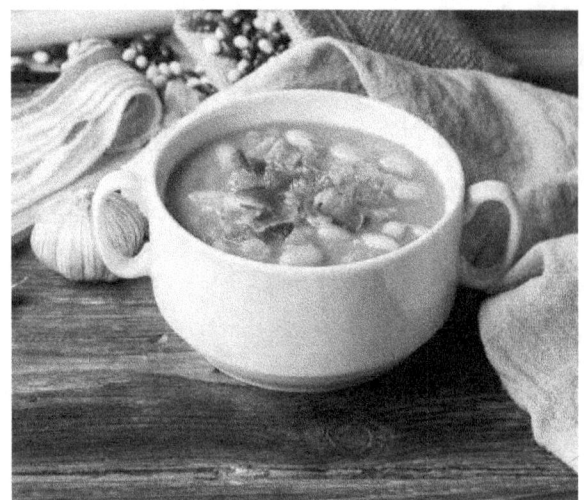

INGREDIENTS

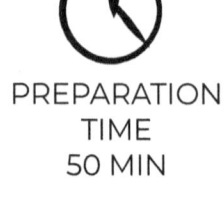

PREPARATION TIME
50 MIN

COOK TIME
3-5 HOUR

SERVING
2

- 1 Cup dried kidney beans
- 1.5 and 2/3 Cups water
- 1.5 Tsp. salt
- 2/3 Cup potato flakes
- ¼ Cup milk
- 1 Tbsp. butter
- ¼ Tsp. salt
- 4 Strips beef jerky

DIRECTIONS

1. Soak your dried beans in 1.5 cups of water and salt overnight. Keep them in the fridge to prevent mold from developing on them.
2. When you are ready to eat, boil your beans for about 1.5 hours, or until done. Top the pot with water as needed, to prevent it from boiling off. (Alternatively, cook dried beans in 6 cups of water in the crockpot until they are done, about 3-5 hours.)
3. Thirty minutes before your beans are done, boil 2/3rd cups of water. Add potato flakes and cook them until they are rehydrated. Remove from heat, add milk, butter, and salt. Let it stand for 10 minutes, then fluff it with a fork.
4. Serve ½ cup beans, ½ cup mashed potatoes, and two slices of beef jerky on each plate. Eat fresh.

Nutritions: Calories: 165 Cal; Protein: 4.2 g; Fiber: 1.2 g; Fat: 10.64 g; Carbs: 13.6 g

Chapter 14. Fruit, Juice, Jam & Jelly Recipes

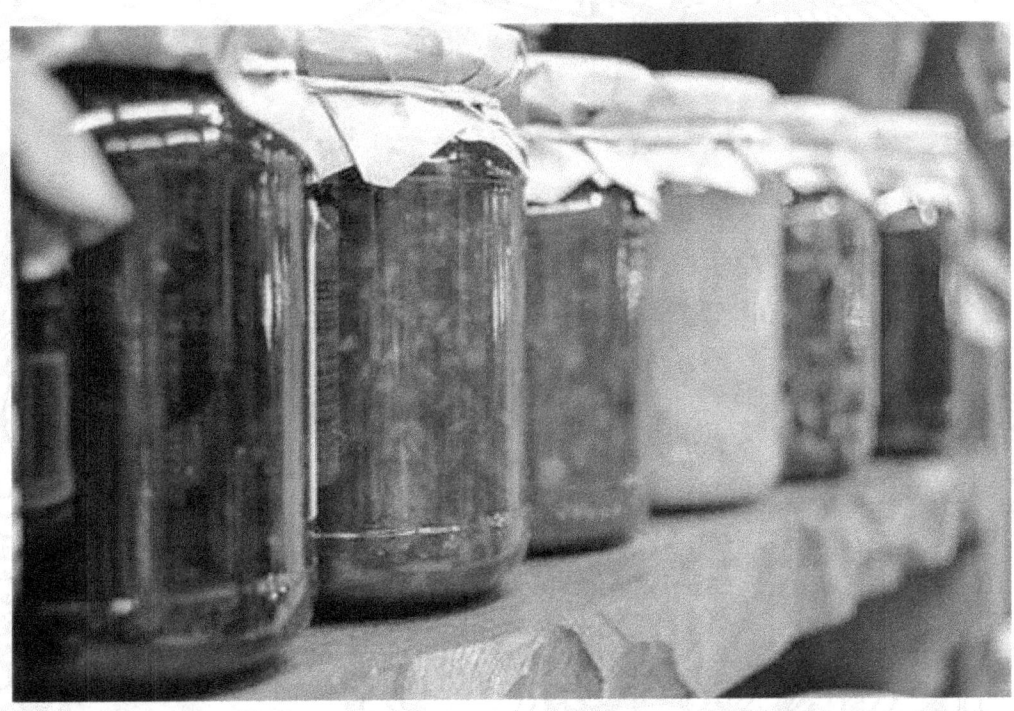

Let's get familiar with all the different categories in terms of preserving. Below you will find a list along with some definitions so you know what is a jam, jelly and or marmalade!

- Preserves: Chunks of, you guessed it, fruit! Steeped in syrup or jelly!
- Conserve: Thick and chewy, this contains typically dried fruits and nuts.
- Jam: Created from thinly cut fruit and made with sugar until the right amount of thickness is created.
- Compote: Fruit stewed or cooked in syrup.
- Chutney: A thick sauce from India that contains fruits, vinegar, sugar, and spices and is used as a condiment.

- Jelly: A soft food product made usually with gelatin or pectin. The key here is pectin, it should be sweet, clear and semisolid.
- Fruit butter: A sweet spread made of fruit cooked to a paste, then lightly sweetened.
- Fruit curd: A dessert spread and topping usually made with citrus fruit
- Marmalade: A bright and citrusy spread that wows the taste buds!

CANNING JUICES AND SYRUPS FOR FRUITS

The following three items are commonly used to can fruit:

- Juice
- Syrup
- Water

Syrup or juice helps fruit maintain its consistency, color and shape. What it doesn't do is prevent fruit from decomposing.

Since the liquid used to preserve fruit doesn't have anything to do with the actual preservation itself, you can experiment a bit with the canning liquid you use for your fruits.

When it comes to syrups, you'll probably want to use a light syrup for sweet fruits. Experiment with the amount of sugar you're using to figure out what tastes best to you.

For tart or sour fruits, you're going to want a heavy syrup. To make a heavier syrup, you're going to need to add more sugar. You can substitute honey for half of the sugar in the chart below for a somewhat healthier syrup.

Use the following chart to figure out how to make the type of syrup you need:

Syrup	Sugar	Sugar
Ultra-Light	1 Cups	1 Cups
Light	2 Cups	2 Cups
Medium	3 Cups	3 Cups
Heavy	4 To 5 Cups	4 To 5 Cups

TIP: *For those who are diabetic, or just don't want to add sugar, artificial sweeteners can be added for additional flavor. Be aware that saccharin and aspartame-based sweeteners don't work well, if added to the canning juice. Add them right before eating the canned fruit for best results.*

Fruit juice can also be used as a canning solution.

Crush ripe fruit and heat it up, then strain it through cheesecloth for best results. The fruit that's being canned is usually the best option. You can also use pineapple, apple or white grape juice.

JAM
53. PINEAPPLE-RHUBARB JAM

Rhubarb is a highly nutritious vegetable that you can process into jam. Combine rhubarb with strawberry gelatin, sugar, water, and pineapple and cook for a few minutes, and the result is an awesome bread spread that you can serve even if pineapple and rhubarb are out of season.

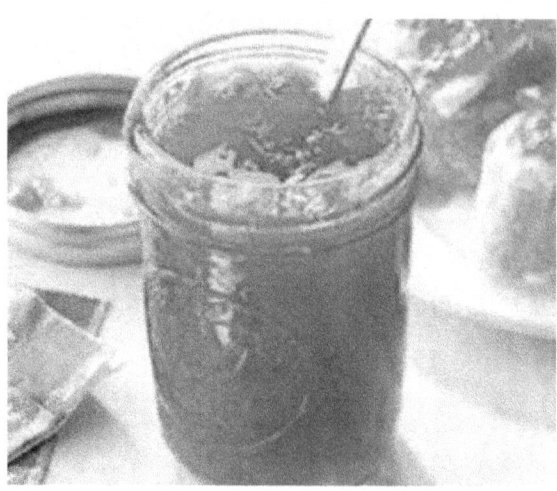

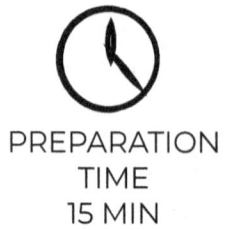

PREPARATION TIME
15 MIN

COOK TIME
20 MIN

SERVING
7 HALF PINT

INGREDIENTS

- 1 (6 ounces) Package strawberry gelatin
- 5 Cups sugar
- 5 Cups (12 stalks) sliced fresh or frozen rhubarb
- 1/4 Cup water
- 1 (20 ounces) can of undrained unsweetened crushed pineapple

DIRECTIONS

1. Combine in a Dutch oven, the sugar, rhubarb, water and pineapple and bring to a boil. Simmer on low heat without cover for eighteen to twenty-two minutes.
2. Stir and cook until the rhubarb has broken down. Stir in gelatin and cook until dissolved. Remove the Dutch oven from heat, skimming off foam.
3. Spoon the hot mixture into half-pint jars with one-fourth inch headspace.
4. Skim off air bubbles, by stirring in a hot mixture and adjust the headspace.
5. Wipe the rims with a paper towel and center the lids on jars, screwing on bands to seal it tightly.
6. Place the jars into the canner filled with simmering water. Pour hot water over the jars to cover them with enough water and bring to a boil.
7. After ten minutes of processing, remove the hot jars and let it cool on a padded surface.
8. Take note that the processing time is at about a 1,000 feet altitude, and 1 minute is added to the processing time with every 1,000 feet of extra altitude.
9. Enjoy!

Nutritions: Calories: 89 Cal; Protein: 0 g; Fiber: 0 g; Fat: 0 g; Carbs: 22 g

54. Honey Blueberry Cobbler Jam

This cobbler jam makes use of apple juice, honey and blueberries to blend with ground cinnamon and vanilla extract. It is sweetened with pectin if you are cutting down on sugar. Add nutmeg for an extra crunchy texture.

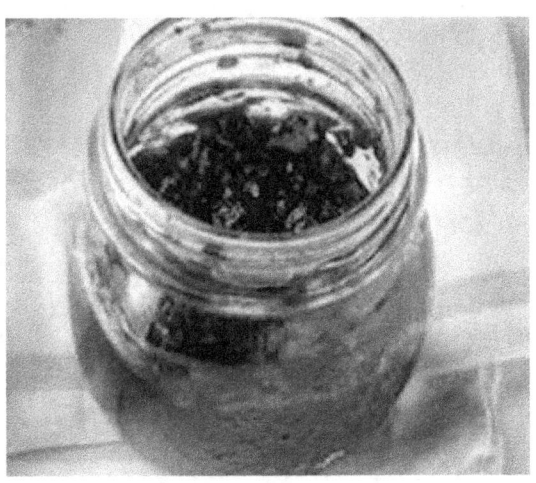

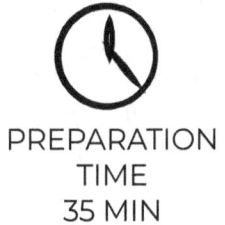
PREPARATION TIME
35 MIN

COOK TIME
24 HOUR

SERVING
5 CUPS

INGREDIENTS

- 1 Cup apple juice
- 5 Cups fresh or thawed frozen blueberries
- 1 Cup honey
- 1/2 Teaspoon ground nutmeg
- 1 Package (1 3/4 ounces) pectin for lower sugar recipes
- 1 Teaspoon vanilla extract
- 1/4 Teaspoon ground cinnamon

DIRECTIONS

1. Prepare blueberries by placing in a large saucepan and mash.
2. Add pectin and juice to mashed blueberries, and bring the mixture to a complete rolling boil on high heat; stirring often to prevent burning.
3. Add nutmeg, honey and cinnamon and place on a full rolling boil, stir frequently for 1 minute.
4. Remove saucepan from the heat and add the vanilla.
5. Rinse five one-cup plastic and lids with hot water, wipe with a paper towel and place the jam with a 1/2 inch headspace.
6. Using a clean dishcloth, wipe off the top edges of plastic containers and cover with lids.
7. Let the jam stand at room temperature for no more than 24 hours.
8. If not using, chill for up to two weeks or freeze for twelve months.
9. When using, thaw frozen jam for an hour in the refrigerator.

Nutritions: Calories: 39 Cal; Protein: 0 g; Fiber: 0 g; Fat: 0 g; Carbs: 10 g

55. Canned Blueberry Jam

Another way to enliven your snacks or brunch is to prepare this jam loaded with fresh blueberries, cinnamon, and sweetened with fruit pectin for less sugary jam and sugar. It is flavored with lemon zest and ground nutmeg for a crunchy texture.

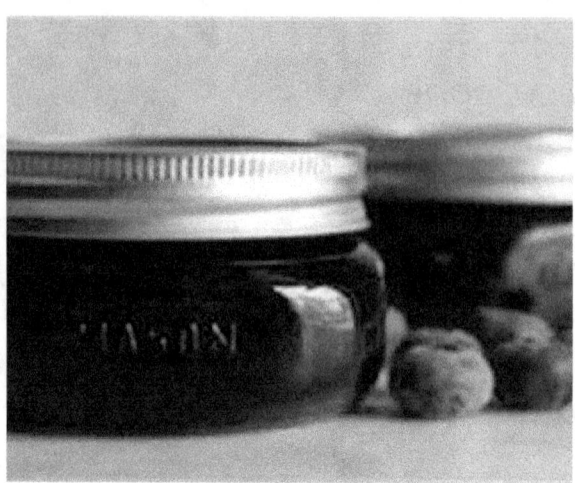

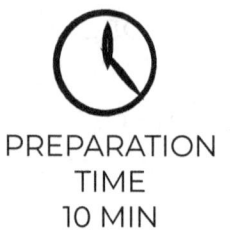
PREPARATION TIME
10 MIN

COOK TIME
15 MIN

SERVING
9 HALF PINTS

INGREDIENTS

- 6 Cups sugar
- 8 Cups fresh blueberries
- 3 Tablespoons lemon juice
- 2 Pouches (3 ounces each) liquid fruit pectin
- 1/2 Teaspoon ground nutmeg
- 2 Teaspoons grated lemon zest
- 2 Teaspoons ground cinnamon

DIRECTIONS

1. Rinse fresh blueberries and place in a food processor; cover and pulse until blended.
2. Pour processed blueberries in a stockpot. Add lemon juice, lemon zest, nutmeg, cinnamon, and sugar to stockpot. Stir and bring to a complete rolling boil on high heat.
3. Sweeten jam with pectin and boil for one minute, stirring often to prevent burning.
4. Remove the stockpot from heat, skimming off foam. Ladle the jam into sterilized half-pint jars and leave at least a ¼ inch headspace.
5. With a plastic knife, remove air bubbles. Wipe the rims with a clean cloth, adjusting the lids before processing for ten minutes in a boiling water canner.
6. Enjoy!

Nutritions: Calories: 74 Cal; Protein: 0 g; Fiber: 0 g; Fat: 0 g; Carbs: 18 g

CONSERVE
56. Victorian Plum Conserve

Scones, toasted bread, or French bread makes a great companion for this homemade spicy conserve, made with the goodness of ripe plums, ripe pears, raisins and navel oranges. Adding a spicy appeal to this spicy conserve is by using cinnamon and allspice, and is sweetened with sugar.

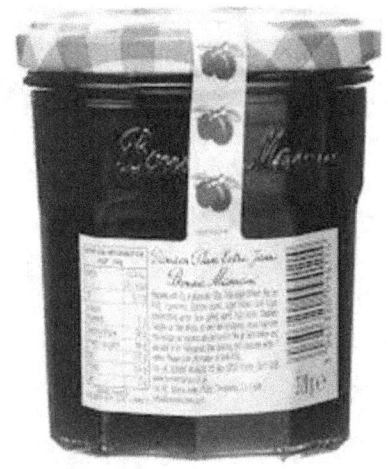

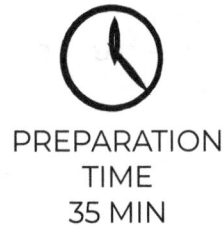

PREPARATION TIME
35 MIN

COOK TIME
1 hour

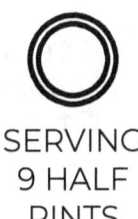

SERVING
9 HALF PINTS

INGREDIENTS

- 12 Ripe plums pitted and coarsely chopped
- 3 Medium navel oranges
- 1/4 Teaspoon ground cinnamon
- 1 Cup chopped peeled ripe pears
- 1 1/2 Cups raisins
- 1/4 Teaspoon ground allspice
- 3 Cups sugar

DIRECTIONS

1. Scrape orange peels and reserve 1/3rd cup of peel. Remove the skin, reject the white membrane and section the flesh.
2. Combine in a large saucepan, the orange sections, orange peel, plums, pears, raisins, cinnamon and allspice; bring to a boil.
3. Simmer on low heat and cook for one hour until it thickens, stirring often.
4. Slowly pour the mixture into the hot, sterile jars with a one-fourth-inch headspace, adjusting the lid, process it for ten minutes in a simmering water bath and bring to a full rolling boil.
5. Serve!

Nutritions: Calories: 51 Cal; Protein: 0 g; Fiber: 0 g; Fat: 0 g; Carbs: 13 g

57. Apple-Walnut Maple Conserve

Your dessert habit will never be the same again with this conserve cooked with the wonders of apple, maple syrup, pumpkin pie spice, toasted walnuts, cinnamon and sweetened with white and brown sugars. It's a great topping for biscuits, ice cream and French toast.

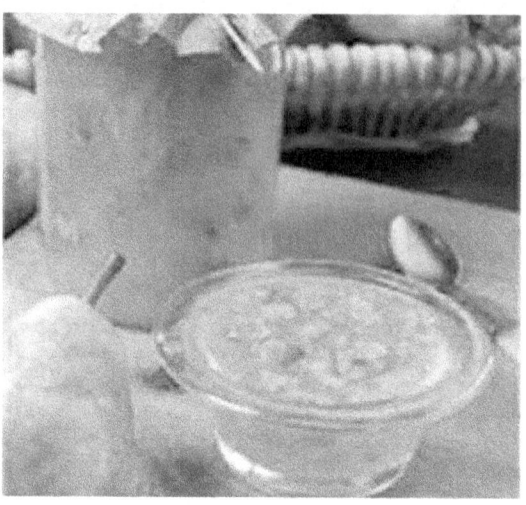

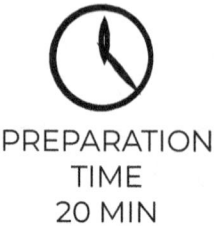

PREPARATION TIME
20 MIN

COOK TIME
50 MIN

SERVING
11 HALF PINTS

INGREDIENTS

- 4 Cups sugar
- 12 Cups chopped peeled Granny Smith apples
- 1 Cup maple syrup
- 2 Cups finely chopped toasted walnuts
- 2 Cups packed brown sugar
- 1 Teaspoon pumpkin pie spice
- 1 Teaspoon ground cinnamon

DIRECTIONS

1. Combine in a stockpot, the apples, maple syrup, pie spice, cinnamon and sugars and bring to a full boil. Cook without cover for twenty to thirty minutes until it is thickened, and the apples have softened.
2. Add walnuts and boil again, stir and cook for five minutes.
3. Slowly ladle the hot conserve into 11 hot half-pint jars, with a ¼ inch headspace, by pouring hot mixture.
4. Wipe the rims with a paper towel, center the lids on the jar, screwing on bands to fingertip tight.
5. Put the jars in simmering water in the canner, and bring it to a complete rolling boil for ten minutes. Remove from the canner and let it cool.
6. Enjoy!

Nutritions: Calories: 89 Cal; Protein: 0 g; Fiber: 0 g; Fat: 2 g; Carbs: 19 g

COMPOTE
58. Cranberry Pear Compote

A great way to spend time together with loved ones is to drink a cup of coffee with French toast or pound cake, topped with this zest-sweet compote. It is a blend of apple, pear, cranberries, and ground cinnamon and sweetened with brown sugar.

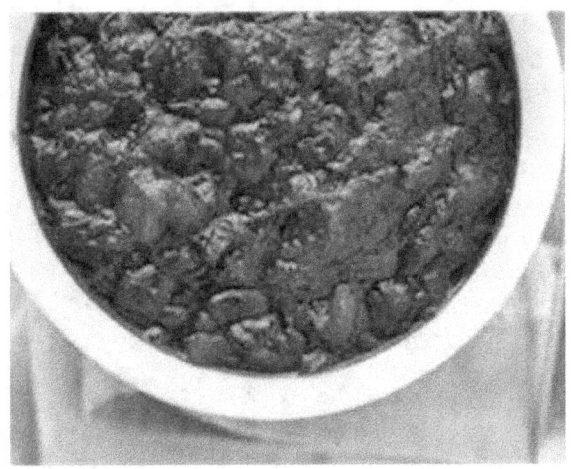

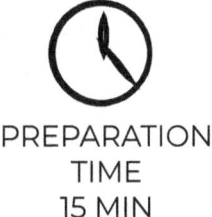

PREPARATION TIME 15 MIN

COOK TIME 15 MIN

INGREDIENTS

- 1 Medium peeled and chopped apple
- 1 Medium peeled and chopped pear
- 1/4 Cup water
- 1/4 Cup fresh or frozen cranberries
- 1/2 Teaspoon ground cinnamon
- 3 Tablespoons brown sugar

SERVING 4

DIRECTIONS

1. Mix all the ingredients in a small saucepan; bring to a full rolling boil.
2. Uncover and simmer over low heat for fifteen minutes until the sauce is consistent and the berries are broken down.
3. Stir and remove from the burner. Place it in sterilized jars and let it cool.
4. Keep refrigerated.
5. Serve!

Nutritions: Calories: 85 Cal; Protein: 0 g; Fiber: 2 g; Fat: 0 g; Carbs: 22 g

59. Delightful Fruit Compote

This fruit compote will definitely receive accolades from your guests during special occasions. You can never get wrong with its delightful fruit compositions, such as blueberries, peaches, kiwifruit, strawberries, and grapes. It tastes so excellent when topped with apple jelly, vanilla yogurt and slice almonds.

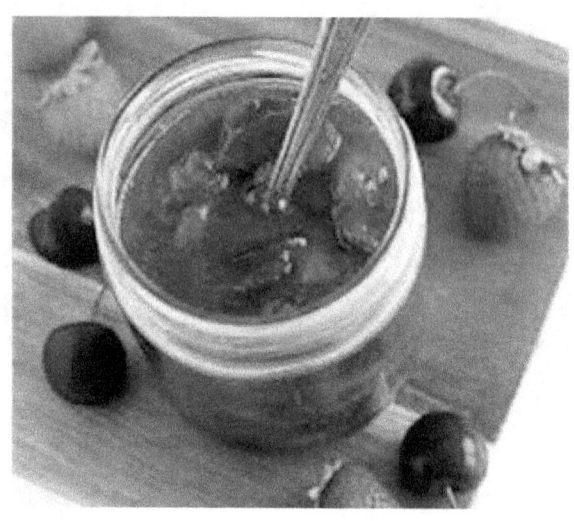

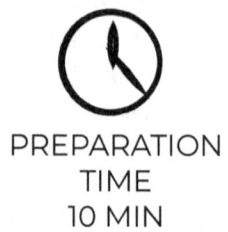

PREPARATION TIME
10 MIN

COOK TIME
15 MIN

SERVING
8

INGREDIENTS

- 1 Cup fresh or frozen blueberries
- 2 Medium sliced ripe peaches
- 2 Kiwifruit, peeled and sliced
- 1 Cup quartered fresh strawberries
- 4 Teaspoons water
- 3 Tablespoons apple jelly
- 3/4 Cup seedless red or green grapes
- Vanilla yogurt and sliced almonds (optional)

DIRECTIONS

1. Combine in a large bowl the berries, peaches, grapes and kiwi, set aside.
2. Mix jelly and water in a heat-proof bowl. Microwave without a cover on high for forty-five seconds until smooth and the jelly has melted.
3. Drizzle mixture over the fruits. Spread yogurt over the jelly mixture and garnish with almonds.
4. Enjoy!

Nutritions: Calories: 80 Cal; Protein: 1 g; Fiber: 2 g; Fat: 0 g; Carbs: 20 g

MARMELADE
60. Quince Orange Marmalade

Skipping breakfast will no longer be a scenario when you prepare your bread with this tangy-sweet marmalade. This marmalade will become part of your daily habit as you can't resist the delicious taste of quince cooked with orange zest and orange juice.

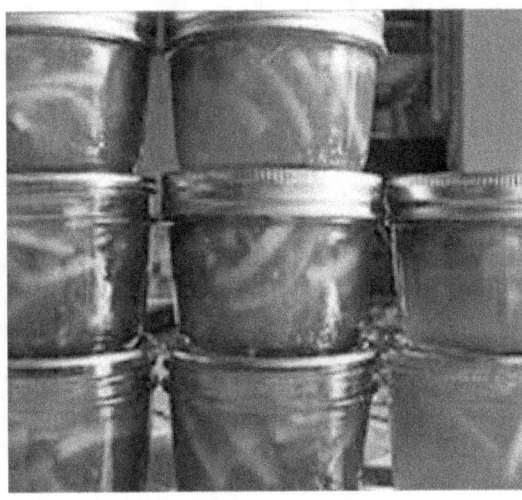

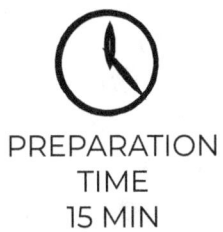
PREPARATION TIME
15 MIN

COOK TIME
15 MIN

SERVING
3 CUPS

INGREDIENTS

- 5 Cups chopped peeled quince
- 1 1/3 Cups sugar
- 1 1/2 Cups water
- 1 Tablespoon grated orange zest
- 1 Cup orange juice

DIRECTIONS

1. Mix in a large saucepan all the ingredients and bring to a boil.
2. Remove the cover and simmer on low heat for 1 ½ to 1 ¾ hours until the sauce is reduced to three cups.
3. Keep stirring to prevent burning. Let it cool slightly and mash.
4. When done, fill jars with a ½ inch allowance from the tops. Wipe off the top edges of jars and cool at room temperature.
5. Keep refrigerated for up to three weeks or frozen for 12 months.
6. Thaw frozen marmalade in the refrigerator and serve with bread.
7. Serve!

Nutritions: Calories: 58 Cal; Protein: 0 g; Fiber: 0 g; Fat: 0 g; Carbs: 15 g

61. Three-Fruit Marmalade

This bread spread got its name from its mixture of three fruits, such as peaches, orange, and pears. It is simply made by cooking in full rolling, boiling it together with fruit pectin and sugar to enhance its fruity taste.

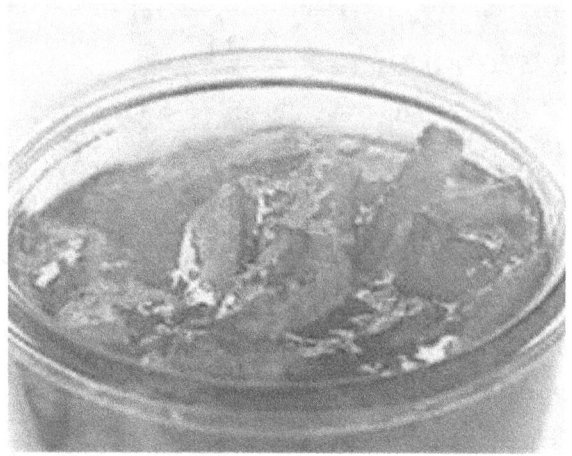

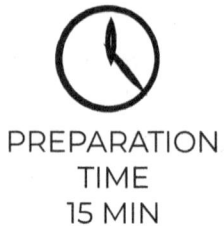

PREPARATION TIME
15 MIN

COOK TIME
15 MIN

SERVING
8 HALF PINTS

INGREDIENTS

- 2 Cups chopped peeled fresh peaches
- 5 Cups sugar
- 1 Medium orange
- 1 Package (1 3/4 ounces) powdered fruit pectin
- 2 Cups chopped peeled fresh pears

DIRECTIONS

1. Grate the orange peel. Peel and section the orange fruit. Put the orange sections and peel in a Dutch oven.
2. Stir in pears, peaches and add the pectin; bring it to a full boil on high heat.
3. Stir often and add the sugar. Return to a complete rolling boil, boil again and stir for one minute.
4. Remove from the burner, skimming off the foam.
5. Ladle the hot marmalade into eight sterilized half-pint jars with one-fourth inch headspace.
6. With a plastic spoon, remove the air bubbles, adjusting headspace by pouring the hot mixture if desired.
7. Wipe the rims with cloth, center the lids on the jars and screw on band up to fingertip tight.
8. Place the jars in the canner with enough simmering water to cover the entire jars.
9. Bring water to a full rolling boil and process for ten minutes. Remove the jars from the canner, and let it cool.
10. Serve!

Nutritions: Calories: 88 Cal; Protein: 0 g; Fiber: 0 g; Fat: 0 g; Carbs: 23 g

62. Orange Pineapple Marmalade

Gift-giving on special occasions could be appreciated if you give the person something you made. What about giving that person this homemade marmalade? This priceless gift will truly be appreciated because it is extra delicious and it comes from the bottom of your heart.

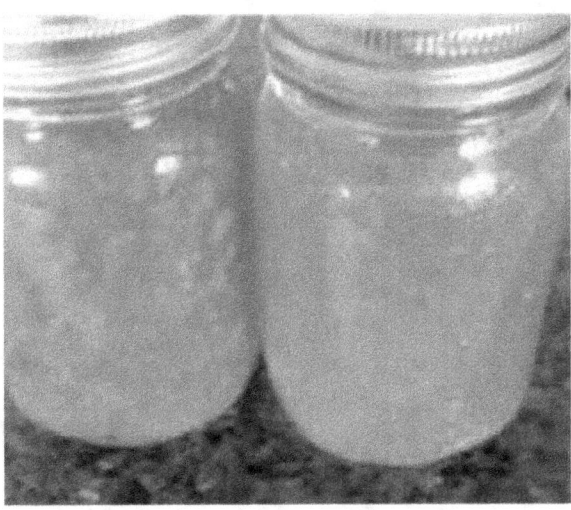

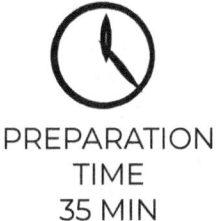

PREPARATION TIME
35 MIN

COOK TIME
1 H 20

SERVING
4 CUPS

INGREDIENTS

- 2 Cans (8 ounces each) drained crushed pineapple
- 2 Medium oranges
- 2 Tablespoons lemon juice
- 4 Cups sugar

DIRECTIONS

1. Wash four one-cup plastic containers and lids, and sterilize them with boiling water. Dry and set aside.
2. Scrape the orange peel, and set aside. Peel off the orange, discarding the white membrane, section the flesh and remove the seeds.
3. Combine in a food processor, the orange sections and zest. Cover and pulse until the orange turns into small bits.
4. Place lemon juice, the orange mixture, sugar and pineapple in a 2 ½ quart microwave safe bowl with a wide bottom.
5. Microwave the mixture without a cover on high for 2 to 2 ½ minutes.
6. Stir and heat until bubbly, stir again and microwave for another 1 ½ to 2 minutes until the middle part is bubbly. Stir and heat for two more minutes, stir often and let cool for ten minutes.
7. Ladle the hot marmalade into plastic containers, leaving a ½ inch allowance from the tops.
8. Wipe off the edges with paper towels. Let it cool for 1 hour. Cover the plastic containers and let it stand for four hours at room temperature.
9. Keep refrigerated for up to three weeks or keep frozen for up to one year.
10. Thaw for an hour or so in the refrigerator before you serve the marmalade.
11. Enjoy!

Nutritions: Calories: 104 Cal; Protein: 0 g; Fiber: 0 g; Fat: 1 g; Carbs: 27 g

63. Pear Marmalade

Although this 'Pear Marmalade' is called this way, it is not going solo on making this as a favorite breakfast companion, since the recipe also calls for pineapple. It is flavored with orange zest, lemon juice and orange juice and sweetened with fruit pectin and sugar.

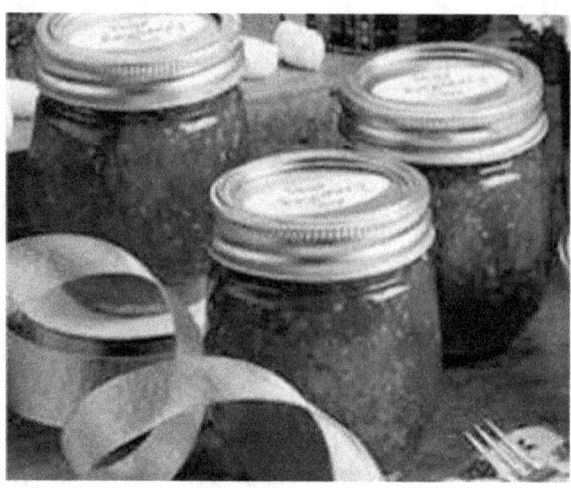

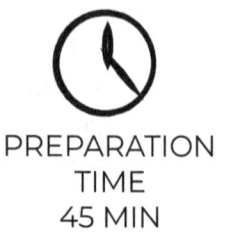

PREPARATION TIME
45 MIN

COOK TIME
24 HOUR

SERVING
6 CUPS

INGREDIENTS

- 1 (8 ounces) Can undrained unsweetened crushed pineapple
- 4-5 Medium peeled and quartered ripe pears
- 2 Tablespoons lemon juice
- 5 1/2 Cups sugar
- 1/2 Cup orange juice
- 1 Package (1 3/4 ounces) powdered fruit pectin
- 1 Tablespoon grated orange zest

DIRECTIONS

1. Place pears in a food processor in batches, and cover and pulse until smooth.
2. Measure out the pears to come up with 1 ½ cups, set aside.
3. Place in a Dutch oven, the lemon juice, pear puree, orange zest, orange juice and pineapple.
4. Add pectin to the fruit mixture and bring it to a complete rolling boil on high heat. Stir often and add the sugar. Boil to full and boil again for 1 minute, stirring frequently.
5. Remove from burner, skimming off foam.
6. Ladle the hot marmalade into jars and let it cool for an hour at room temperature.
7. Let it stand with cover for a maximum of 24 hours until completely set. Chill for up to three weeks or keep frozen for one year.
8. Enjoy!

Nutritions: Calories: 101 Cal; Protein: 0 g; Fiber: 0 g; Fat: 0 g; Carbs: 26 g

64. Tomato Lemon Marmalade

This marmalade is high in nutrients with the fusion of tomatoes, apples, lemons, gingers and cloves. Its tangy-zesty aroma will surely make you want for more than a slice of bread. If you want it less sugary, you can lessen the sugar and add fruit pectin instead.

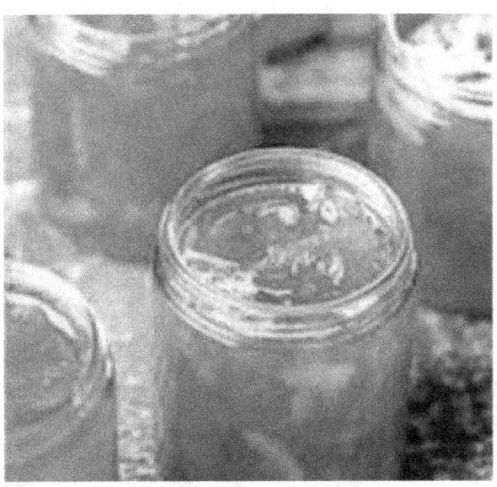

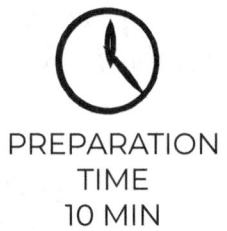
PREPARATION TIME
10 MIN

COOK TIME
20 MIN

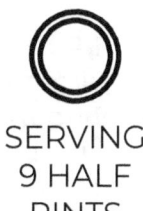
SERVING
9 HALF PINTS

INGREDIENTS

- 4 Cups (4 apples) chopped peeled tart apples
- 5 Medium ripe tomatoes
- 6 Cups sugar
- 2 Medium seeded and finely chopped lemons
- 8 Whole cloves
- 2 1/4 Teaspoons ground ginger

DIRECTIONS

1. Prepare the tomatoes by peeling them, slicing them into quarters and then chopping them.
2. Place chopped tomatoes in a colander to drain before placing in a Dutch oven.
3. Add the lemons and apples to the Dutch oven, cook for fifteen minutes on moderate heat, stirring often. Stir in ginger and sugar.
4. Place cloves in cheesecloth bag and tie; add to the mixture.
5. Bring the mixture to a complete rolling boil; stirring often, and cook until the sugar has melted. Simmer on low for forty minutes, stirring frequently.
6. Discard the spice bag and ladle the hot marmalade into nine sterilized hot half-pint jars with a 1/4 inch headspace.
7. Remove the air bubbles with a plastic knife, adjusting the headspace and wipe the rims, center the lids on the jars and screw them on the bands.
8. Place the jars into the canner with simmering water, just enough to cover it; bring to a full boil, and process it for ten minutes.
9. Remove the jars and place them on a padded work surface. Let it cool.
10. Enjoy!

Nutritions: Calories: 142 Cal; Protein: 0 g; Fiber: 1 g; Fat: 0 g; Carbs: 36 g

65. Mixed Citrus Marmalade

Bagels, French toast, or bread rolls will taste better if you slather this tangy-sweet marmalade. It is a combined effort of lemons, grapefruit and oranges plus a cup of brewed coffee to boost your brunch or breakfast.

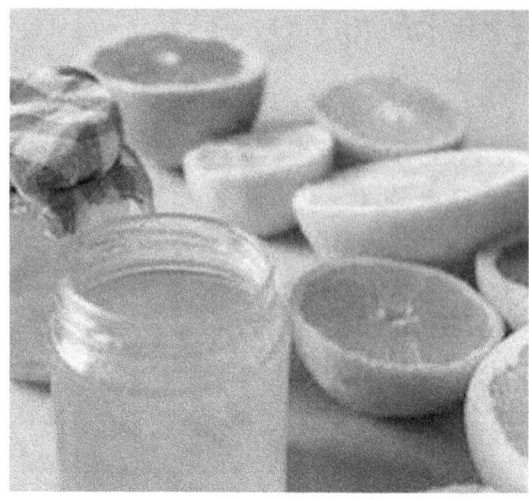

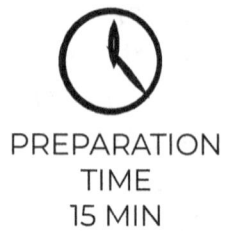

PREPARATION TIME
15 MIN

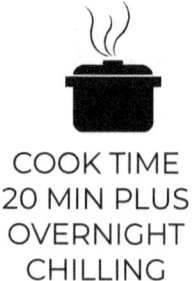

COOK TIME
20 MIN PLUS OVERNIGHT CHILLING

SERVING
10 HALF PINTS

INGREDIENTS

- 1 Pound Oranges, thinly sliced and seeds removed
- 1 Pound Grapefruit, thinly sliced and seeds removed
- 1 Pound Lemons, thinly sliced and seeds removed
- 8 Cups sugar
- 2 Quarts water

DIRECTIONS

1. Combine in a large mixing bowl the oranges, grapefruit, lemons and 2 quarts water; cover and chill overnight.
2. Place the fruit mixture in a Dutch oven; bring to a complete rolling boil. Remove cover; simmer on low heat for about ten to fifteen minutes until tender.
3. Add the sugar, stir and boil. Cook for forty to fifty-five minutes, stirring often until thickened.
4. Remove from the burner and skim off the foam.
5. Slowly ladle the hot marmalade into sterilized half-pint jars with a one-fourth inch headspace.
6. Remove the air bubbles using a plastic spoon.
7. Wipe the rims, adjust the lids and process for five minutes in a canner filled with boiling water. Remove from heat, and let it cool.
8. Serve!

Nutritions: Calories: 82 Cal; Protein: 0 g; Fiber: 0 g; Fat: 0 g; Carbs: 82 g

66. Strawberry Marmalade

When strawberries are in abundance, the best way that you can preserve them is by following this recipe. This tangy-fruity marmalade is made possible by combining the oranges, lemons and strawberries and sweetened by adding pectin and sugar. Baking soda is also added as a thickener.

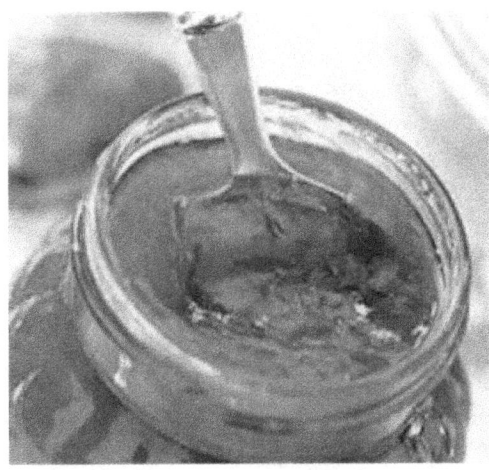

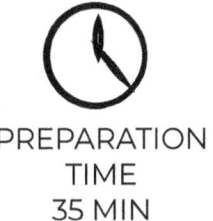
PREPARATION TIME 35 MIN

COOK TIME 50 MIN

SERVING 10 HALF PINTS

INGREDIENTS

- 2 Medium lemons
- 2 Medium oranges
- 1/8 Teaspoon baking soda
- 1 Pouch (6 ounces) liquid fruit pectin
- 1/2 Cup water
- 7 Cups sugar
- 1 Quart crushed ripe strawberries

DIRECTIONS

1. Remove the outer layer of lemons and oranges. Remove the fruits' white membrane and discard them.
2. Chop the fruit peels and put them in a saucepan. Pour ½ cup of water and add the baking soda. Cover and boil, reduce the heat and simmer for ten minutes.
3. Section the lemons and oranges, reserve the juice; add to the saucepan. Cover and simmer on low heat for twenty minutes. Stir in strawberries.
4. Measure out the fruit to come up with four cups and place it in the pan, discarding the excess.
5. Stir in sugar and boil it uncovered, for five minutes. Add pectin and boil it for one minute, stirring frequently.
6. Remove from the burner and skim off the foam. Cautiously ladle the hot marmalade into ten hot sterilized half-pint jars, leaving an allowance of ¼ inch headspace.
7. Remove any air bubbles with a plastic knife, adjusting the headspace.
8. Wipe the rims, center the lids on the jars, and screw on the bands.
9. Place the jars in boiling water in the canner, boil and process for ten minutes. Remove the jars and let cool.
10. Enjoy!

Nutritions: Calories: 71 Cal; Protein: 0 g; Fiber: 0 g; Fat: 0 g; Carbs: 18 g

67. Jalapeño Pepper Jelly

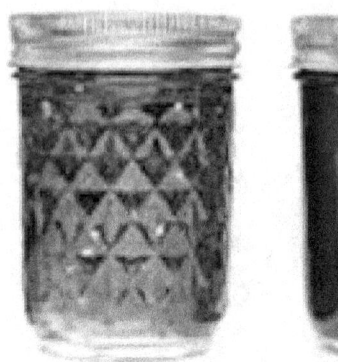
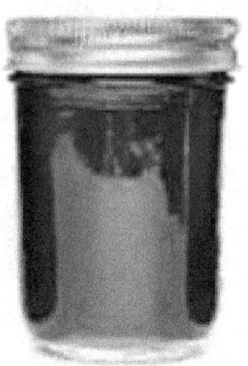

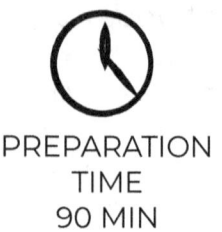

PREPARATION TIME
90 MIN

COOK TIME
20 MIN

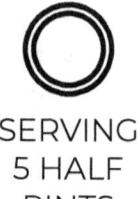

SERVING
5 HALF PINTS

INGREDIENTS

- 1 Cup, chopped green bell pepper
- 1/3 Cup of chopped jalapeño pepper
- 4 Cups of sugar
- 1 Cup of cider vinegar
- 1 Packet of pectin, about 6 ounces

DIRECTIONS

1. Mix all the ingredients together in a large saucepot, and let it boil for about five minutes.
2. Next, let it cool to room temperature for about one hour, and then put them into jars.
3. Let the jars sit in a water bath for five minutes, and then let them sit at room temperature for about twelve to 24 hours before storing.

Nutritions: Calories: 651 Cal; Fat: 26 g; Carbs: 93 g; Protein: 17 g; Sodium: 112 mg

68. Just Jalapeno Blackberry Jelly

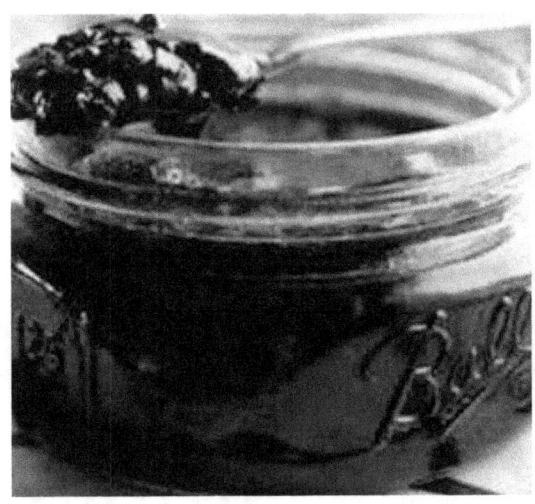

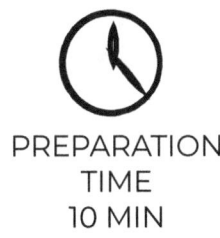

PREPARATION TIME
10 MIN

COOK TIME
40 MIN

SERVING
5

INGREDIENTS

- ½ Cup white sugar
- 1 Pack of 1.75 oz. powdered pectin
- 4 Cups blackberry juice
- 1 Red jalapeno pepper, minced
- 1 Green jalapeno pepper, minced
- 3 ½ Cups white sugar

DIRECTIONS

1. In a bowl, mix in the sugar (1/2 cup) and pectin crystals.
2. To make the jelly, take a heavy saucepan; mix in the jalapeno (both), pectin mixture and blackberry juice.
3. Keep the heat on a medium setting; let the mixture heat for a few minutes.
4. Then mix in the sugar (3 ½ cups) and continue heating until it dissolves completely.
5. After that, remove it from the heat; remove the foam using a spoon.
6. Then take the pre-sterilized jars; place the blackberry jelly mixture into the jars.
7. Keep a ½ inch margin from the top.
8. Use a damp cloth to clean jar rims; then close them with the lid and band.
9. Afterwards, place the jars in the canning pot filled with water.
10. Set the canning timer at 5-7 minutes; adjust the canning time based on your altitude level.
11. After the canning time is over, take out the hot jars, wipe them and take off the bands.
12. Store in a dry, cool place and enjoy the delicious jelly!

Nutritions: Calories: 690 Cal; Fat: 19 g; Carbs: 114 g; Protein: 21 g; Sodium 166 mg

69. Savory Ruby Port Vinegar Jelly

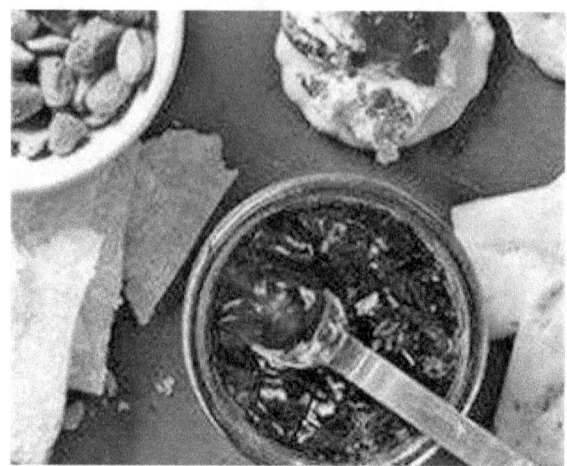

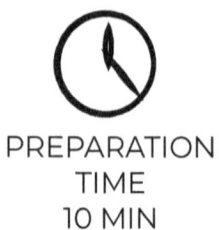

PREPARATION TIME
10 MIN

COOK TIME
30 MIN

SERVING
4

INGREDIENTS

- ¼ Cup orange peel, shredded
- 1/3 Cup balsamic vinegar
- 3 Cups sugar
- 1 Pack of 3 oz. liquid fruit pectin
- 2 Cups ruby port

DIRECTIONS

1. To make the jelly, take a heavy saucepan; mix in the orange peel and vinegar.
2. Keep the heat on a medium setting; let the mixture heat for about 4-5 minutes.
3. Remove the peel from the hot mixture.
4. Place the vinegar mixture back in the saucepan and add the port and sugar.
5. Keep the heat on a high setting; then add in the pectin and continue boiling for about 1-2 more minutes.
6. Then remove it from the heat; remove the foam using a spoon.
7. After that take the pre-sterilized jars; place the jelly mixture into the jars.
8. Keep a ½ inch margin from the top.
9. Use a damp cloth to clean jar rims; then close them with the lid and band.
10. Afterwards, place the jars in the canning pot filled with water.
11. Set the canning timer at 10 minutes; adjust the canning time based on your altitude level.
12. After the canning time is over, take out the hot jars, wipe them and take off the bands.
13. Store in a dry, cool area and enjoy the delicious jelly.

Nutritions: Calories: 651 Cal; Fat: 26 g; Carbs: 93 g; Protein: 17 g; Sodium 112 mg

70. Rosy Jelly Retreat

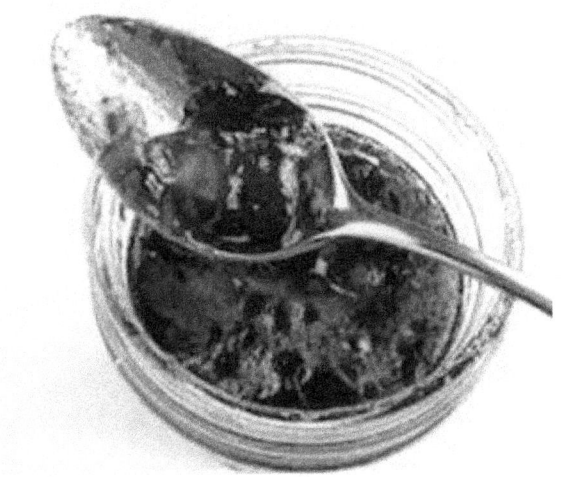

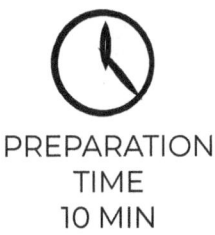

PREPARATION TIME
10 MIN

COOK TIME
25 MIN

SERVING
7

INGREDIENTS

- 3 ¼ Cups white sugar
- ¾ Cup grape juice
- 2 Cups cranberry juice
- 1 Pack of 2 oz. dry pectin

DIRECTIONS

1. To make the jelly, take a heavy cooking pot; mix in the pectin and both grape and cranberry juices in it.
2. Keep the heat on a medium setting; let the mixture heat for few minutes.
3. Mix in the sugar; stir the mixture and let it dissolve completely.
4. After that, remove it from the heat; remove the foam using a spoon.
5. Then take the pre-sterilized jars; place the grape jelly mixture into the jars.
6. Keep a ½ inch margin from the top.
7. Use a damp cloth to clean jar rims; then close them with the lid and band.
8. Afterwards, place the jars in the canning pot filled with water.
9. Set the canning timer at 10 minutes; adjust the canning time based on your altitude level.
10. After the canning time is over, take out the hot jars, wipe them and take off the bands.
11. Store in a dry, cool area and enjoy the delicious grape jelly!

Nutritions: Calories: 690 Cal; Fat: 19 g; Carbs: 114 g; Protein: 21 g; Sodium 166 mg

CONCLUSION

I would like to thank you for taking the time to buy this book and read the content of this work. I hope that you found recipes that you loved, and that you will have a lot of fun trying out each and every one of them.
Canning and preserving are somewhat of an exact science. Follow the recipes exactly, and you will be fine. The pointers and tips in this work were meant to help you become more of a pro with canning food. I hope you will soon be comfortable and capable of the basic process of canning. You'll even be creating concoctions of your own!
Canning and pickling are quite a fruitful hobby, and a great way to store food in your pantry. You are not only harboring an eco-friendly hobby, but avoiding processed food alternatives, which have been preserved with unnatural means, to begin with.
Canning your own food is a deeply satisfying activity. When you take a look at your canned foods and you realize that you were able to do it on your own, it will fuel the motivation for you to turn this into a regular habit. If you choose to can your own food on a regular basis, you will notice a decline in the amount of money you use to buy produce and other canned foods. Home canning will also influence your eating habits in a positive way. The foods you will preserve will be far healthier than the preserved foods that are sold in the supermarkets.

Once you get the hang of canning your own food, you will be unstoppable! I will not lie to you and tell you that everything will be easy, especially the first couple of times. You will make a couple of mistakes and you might make a mess of your kitchen too. This is expected; you are a beginner after all.

As time goes by, though, the number of mistakes you make will decrease and eventually, you won't need this guide to assist you. You will be able to come up with creative recipes of your own! This all has to start with the first steps, the first steps being, you giving this a chance.

Don't let your fears stop you from trying out this great method of preserving your own food. It is a highly rewarding experience that is capable of benefitting you for years to come.
You won't regret trying it out!

APPENDIX

APPENDIX A
Altitudes of Cities in the United States and Canada

UNITED STATES			
State	City	Feet	Meters
Arizona	Mesa	1,243	379
	Phoenix	1,150	351
	Scottsdale	1,257	383
	Tucson	2,389	728
California	Fontana	1,237	377
	Moreno Valley	1,631	497
Colorado	Aurora	5,471	1,668
	Colorado Springs	6,010	1,832
	Denver	5,183	1,580
Georgia	Atlanta	1,026	313
Idaho	Boise	2,730	832
	Idaho Falls	4,705	1,434
Iowa	Sioux City	1,201	366
Kansas	Wichita	1,299	396
Montana	Billings	3,123	952
	Missoula	3,209	978
Nebraska	Lincoln	1,176	358
	Omaha	1,090	332

	Henderson	1,867	569
Nevada	Las Vegas	2,001	610
	Reno	4,505	1,373
New Mexico	Albuquerque	5,312	1,619
	Santa Fe	7,260	2,213
North Carolina	Asheville	2,134	650

UNITED STATES

State	City	Feet	Meters
North Dakota	Bismarck	1,686	514
Ohio	Akron	1,004	306
Oklahoma	Oklahoma City	1,201	366
Pennsylvania	Pittsburgh	1,370	418
South Dakota	Rapid City	3,202	976
Texas	Amarillo	3,605	1,099
	El Paso	3,740	1,140
	Lubbock	3,256	992
Utah	Provo	4,551	1,387
	Salt Lake City	4,226	1,288
Washington	Spokane	1,843	562
Wyoming	Casper	5,150	1,570

CANADA

Province	City	Feet	Meters
Alberta	Calgary	3,600	1,100
	Edmonton	2,201	671
Ontario	Hamilton	1,063	324
Manitoba	Brandon	1,343	409
Saskatchewan	Regina	1,893	577
	Saskatoon	1,580	482

Note: You might use an altimeter or a mobile app on your phone to know the exact altitude of the place you are. That may be the easiest and most accurate method.

APPENDIX B
Food Reference Chart

Type of Food	Pint Processing Time	Quart Processing Time	Headspace
Asparagus	30 minutes	40 minutes	1 inch
Beans, Lima	40 minutes	50 minutes	1-1.5 inches
Beans, Green	20 minutes	25 minutes	1 inch
Beets	30 minutes	35 minutes	1 inch
Carrots	25 minutes	30 minutes	1 inch
Corn kernels	55 minutes	85 minutes	1 inch
Peas	40 minutes	50 minutes	1 inch
Peppers	35 minutes	40 minutes	1 inch
Potatoes	35 minutes	40 minutes	1 inch
Pumpkin	55 minutes	90 minutes	1 inch
Spinach and other greens	70 minutes	90 minutes	1 inch
Vegetable soups	60 minutes	75 minutes	1 inch
Ground meat	75 minutes	90 minutes	1 inch
Meat Strips, cubes or chunks	75 minutes	90 minutes	1 inch
Poultry without bones	75 minutes	90 minutes	1 ¼ inch
Poultry with bones	65 minutes	75 minutes	1 ¼ inch
Meat soups	75 minutes	90 minutes	1 inch
Meat stock	20 minutes	25 minutes	1 inch
Fish	100 minutes	110 minutes	1 inch
Okra	25 minutes	40 minutes	1 inch

Canning and Preserving for Beginners

Pressure Table

Gauge Type	Altitude	Meats & Veggies Pressure	Fruits Required Pressure
Weighted	0-1000 ft.	10 pounds	5 pounds
	1000-8000 ft.	15 pounds	10 pounds
Dial	0-2000 ft.	11 pounds	5 pounds
	2000-4000 ft.	12 pounds	6 pounds
	4000-6000 ft.	13 pounds	7 pounds
	6000-8000 ft.	14 pounds	8 pounds

Fruit Chart

*Note: Headspace for all fruit cooked in a pressure canner is ½ inch.

Fruit	Pint & Quart Minutes
Apples	8 minutes
Applesauce	5 minutes
Berries	8 minutes
Cherries	8 minutes
Cranberries	8 minutes
Figs	10 minutes
Grapes	8 Minutes
Peaches	8 minutes
Pears	8 minutes
Persimmons	10 minutes
Pineapple	8 minutes
Plums	8 minutes
Prunes	8 minutes
Quinces	12 minutes
Raspberries	8 minutes
Rhubarb	5 minutes
Strawberries	5 minutes

| Tomatoes | 10 minutes |
| Fruit juices | 5 minutes |

APPENDIX C
Measurement Conversion Tables

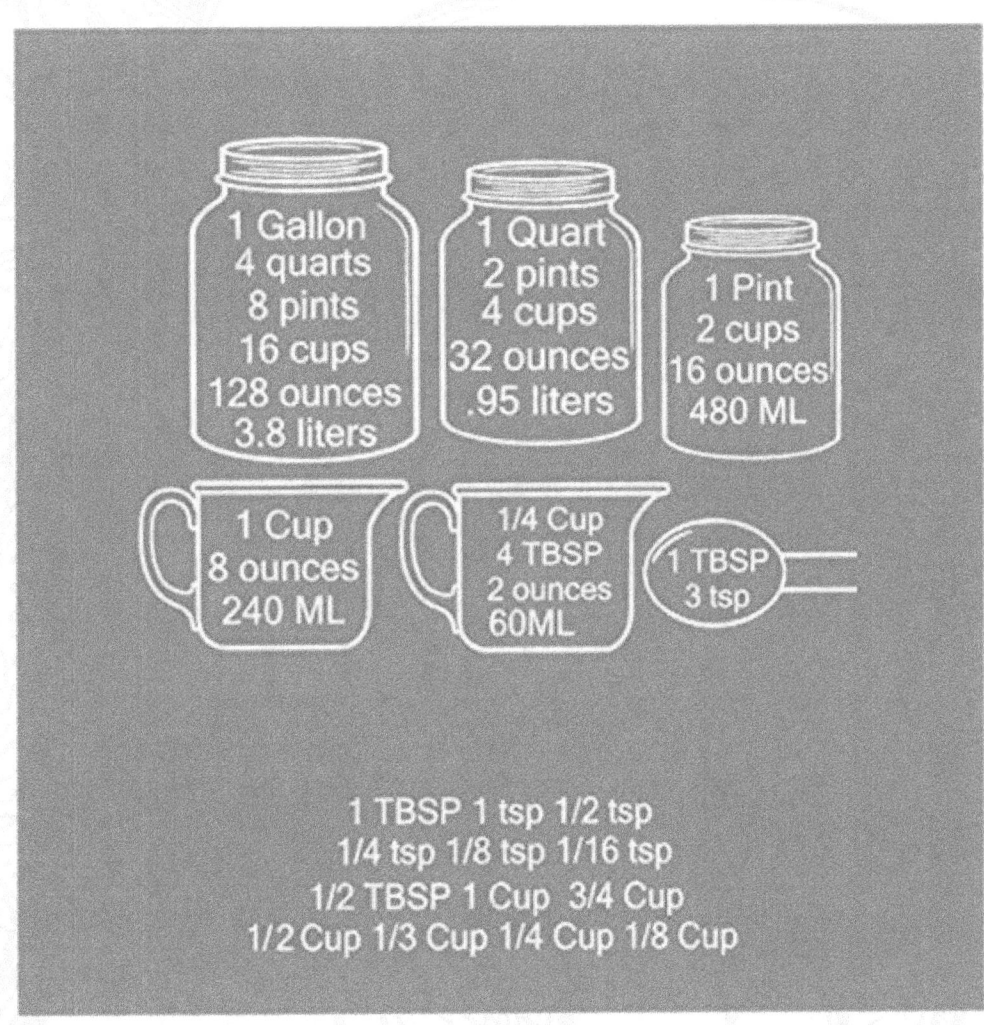

www.ingramcontent.com/pod-product-compliance
Lightning Source LLC
Chambersburg PA
CBHW081359070526
44583CB00020B/2593